FAMILY TREE SECRETS!

Diseases that Tend to Run in Families

Prevalence of a Disease According to Gender, Race, and Genes

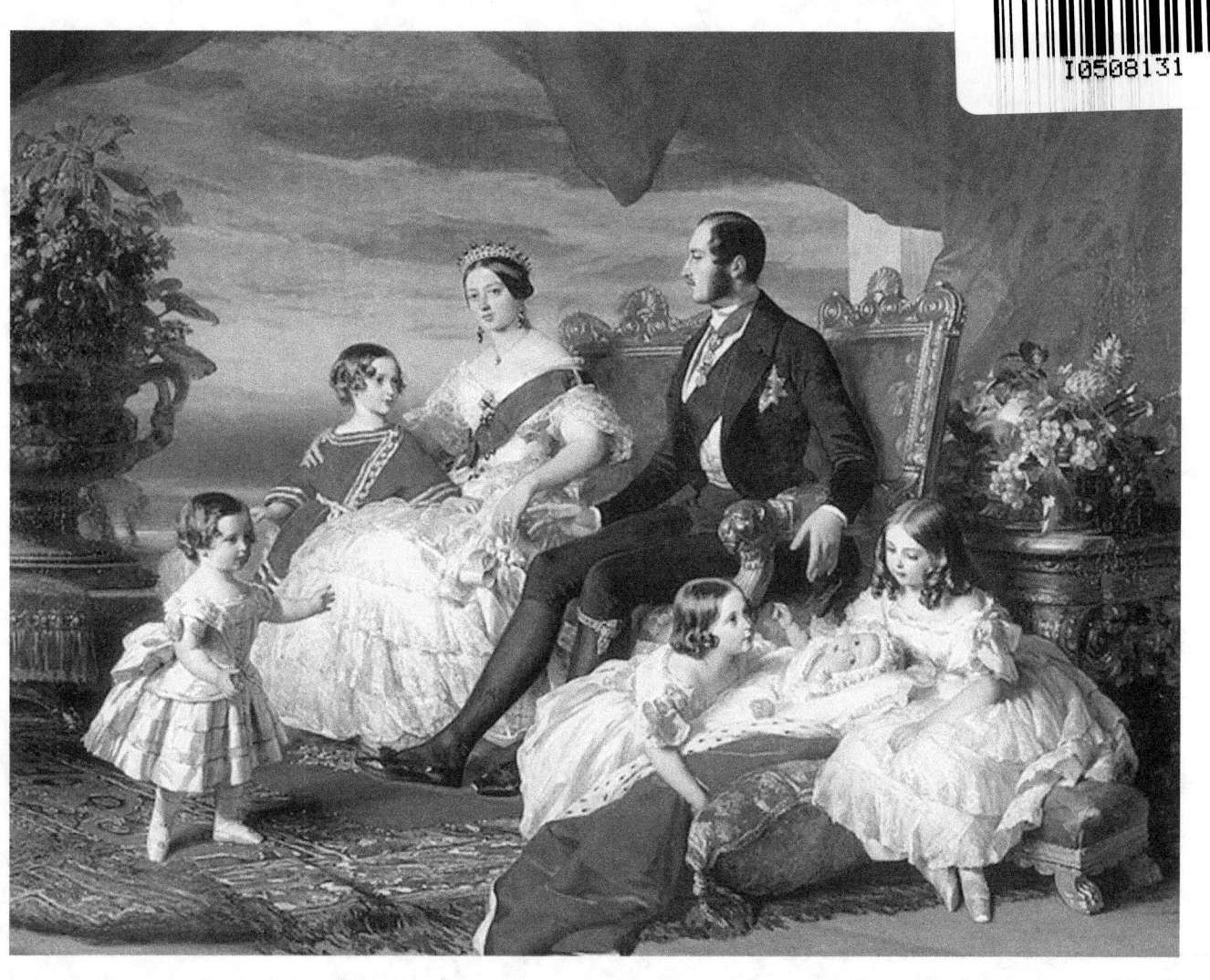

Dr. Ayman Elhossiny, MD

© 2020 Dr. Ayman Elhossiny

All Rights Reserved

ISBN: 9798677248337

CONTENTS

INTRODUCTION	1
DEFINITIONS	2
HEMOPHILIA: THE DISEASE OF EUROPEAN ROYAL FAMILIES	5
HERE IS AMERICA: ARE YOU WHITE, BLACK OR RED	11
WHAT IS SICKLE CELL ANEMIA?	14
AMERICA RANKS FIRST IN DIABETES	17
PANCREATIC CANCER AT A HIGH PERCENTAGE AMONG BLACK AMERICANS	21
CORONAVIRUS SPREAD AMONG BLACKS	24
FACTORS PROMOTING SKIN CANCER	25
WHY AMERICANS ARE MORE SUSCEPTIBLE TO DIVERTICULOSIS?	28
BLUE AMERICANS	34
IS HIGH CHOLESTEROL HEREDITARY?	36
GOUT … IS IT A MALE'S DISEASE?!	40
WHY DO BLADDER INFLAMMATION AND BURNING URINATION PROBLEMS PREVAIL AMONG WOMEN MORE THAN MEN?!	44
WHEN DOES THE CHANCES INCREASE FOR CONTRACTING THE MEDITERRANEAN ANEMIA?	47
WHO ARE THOSE MOST SUSCEPTIBLE TO THE MEDITERRANIAN FEVER?	51
DIFFICULTIES OF THE THYROID, THE WOMEN'S FRIEND!	53
FACTORS THAT ENHANCE THE LIKELIHOOD OF GALLBLADER TROUBLES	57
WHY FEMALES ARE MORE SUSCIPTIBLE TO OSTEOPOROSIS?	60
WHEN DOES THE CHANCE FOR HAVING RHEUMATOID DISEASE INCREASE?	64
WHEN DOES THE CHANCE OF CONCEIVING A CHILD WITH DOWN SYNDROM INCREASE?	68
WHAT ARE THE CHANCES OF ACQUISITION OF BREAST CANCER?	71
SPLIT OF THE AORTA, IS IT RELATED TO A HERIDETATY DEFECT	75
HUNTINGTON DISEASE … IS THE INVOLUNTARY MUSCLE MOVEMENTS HERIDITARY?	79
WHY SOME PEOPLE ARE BALD AND OTHERS ARE NOT?	83
IS OBESITY HEREDITARY?	87
BIPOLAR DISORDER … DO WE INHERIT DEPRESSION AND MANIA EPISODES?	90
HEREDITARY MUSCULAR WEAKNESS (DUCHENNE MUSCULAR DYSTROPHY)	94
DOES PARKINSON DISEASE PREVAIL IN FAMILIES?	97
HEREDITARY FAVA BEANS ANEMIA	100
HEREDITARY PROTEIN DISEASE (PKU)	104
CHANCES OF CONTRACTING ASHKENAZI JEWS DISEASES	107

INTRODUCTION

How does a disease select its victims? Regardless of the environmental factors and the different lifestyles that provide ample opportunities for the disease to strike and gets someone sick, there are factors that beyond our control that gets someone specific sick. Some diseases may prefer females, others are more biased to males. In other words, the sex factor plays a role in contracting some diseases. A disease may spread among certain breed while another is more spread among another breed. A disease may be associated with one family or race while other races are likely to be victims of a different types of diseases. Undoubtedly, the variation of genetics among humans, generally plays a major role in being prone to specific diseases according to what the heredity genes carry from information, abilities and traits that are common or specific.

Accordingly, tracing the hereditary disease in the family tree could be of value in assessing the possibility of contracting a specific disease. If one cannot change or control our sex, race, or genetic makeup to avoid contracting specific diseases, one can oftentimes identify the chances of development of some disease, whether through genetic examination or through the avoidance of the factors that maximizes the opportunity of contracting those diseases or passing a hereditary disease to our offsprings. One possible way is to avoid marrying close relations.

This is the topic of this treatise which presents a genre of diseases that are common and less common which have been acknowledged as being affected by the sex, race, and genetics. The cases are selected form all around the world.

The Author

DEFINITIONS

The word *chromosome* comes from the Greek *chroma* that means "color" and *soma*, that means "body". Accordingly, *chroma soma* refers to colored body or stained body, describing the strong staining of chromosomes by particular dyes.

A chromosome is a DNA (deoxyribonucleic acid) molecule with part or all of the genetic material (genome) of an organism. Most eukaryotic chromosomes include packaging proteins which, aided by chaperone proteins, bind to and condense the DNA molecule to prevent it from becoming an unmanageable tangle. This three-dimensional genome structure plays a significant role in transcriptional regulation.

The chromosomes are present in all living organisms with different numbers. In each human cell, there is 23 pairs of chromosomes (46 chromosomes).

There are two types of chromosomes: body chromosomes (autosomes) that amounts to 22 pairs which contains two types of chromosomes (XY). These chromosomes are responsible for inherited features such as the color of the eyes, height, etc. The other pair is the sex-chromosomes which dictate the gender. The male carries different chromosomes (XY) while the female carries a pair of the same chromosome (X) only; that is (XX). When the cells divide to form the sperm and the ovum, they produce a sperm that contains an X chromosome or Y chromosome, while the ovum contains X chromosomes only. Accordingly, if a sperm of the Y type fertilizes an ovum X the outcome will be male (XY), while a sperm that contains X chromosome fertilizes the ovum it provides a female. In other words, the male is responsible for determination of the gender of a newborn.

The chromosomes contain genes, which are part of the DNA and it carries commands related to building and spiting cells. Genes are the hereditary building blocks that are transferred from parents to offsprings and from one generation to the next. Some chromosomes carry thousands of genes.

Gene mutation means changes in the hereditary commands. An example of gene mutation is the case when cells abnormally undergo rapid divisions leading to the formation of abnormal cells or cancer.

Most hereditary diseases are connected to the genes and only a few are connected to the chromosomes, such as the case when the number of chromosomes is 47 instead of 46. That is the case of the Down syndrome.

The genes are connected to the inherited traits. There is a dominant trait which is the strong characteristic that appears in the offspring whether it is combined with similar or dissimilar characteristics. There is also recessive trait which is the weak characteristic that does not appear in the offspring unless it is combined with a similar trait.

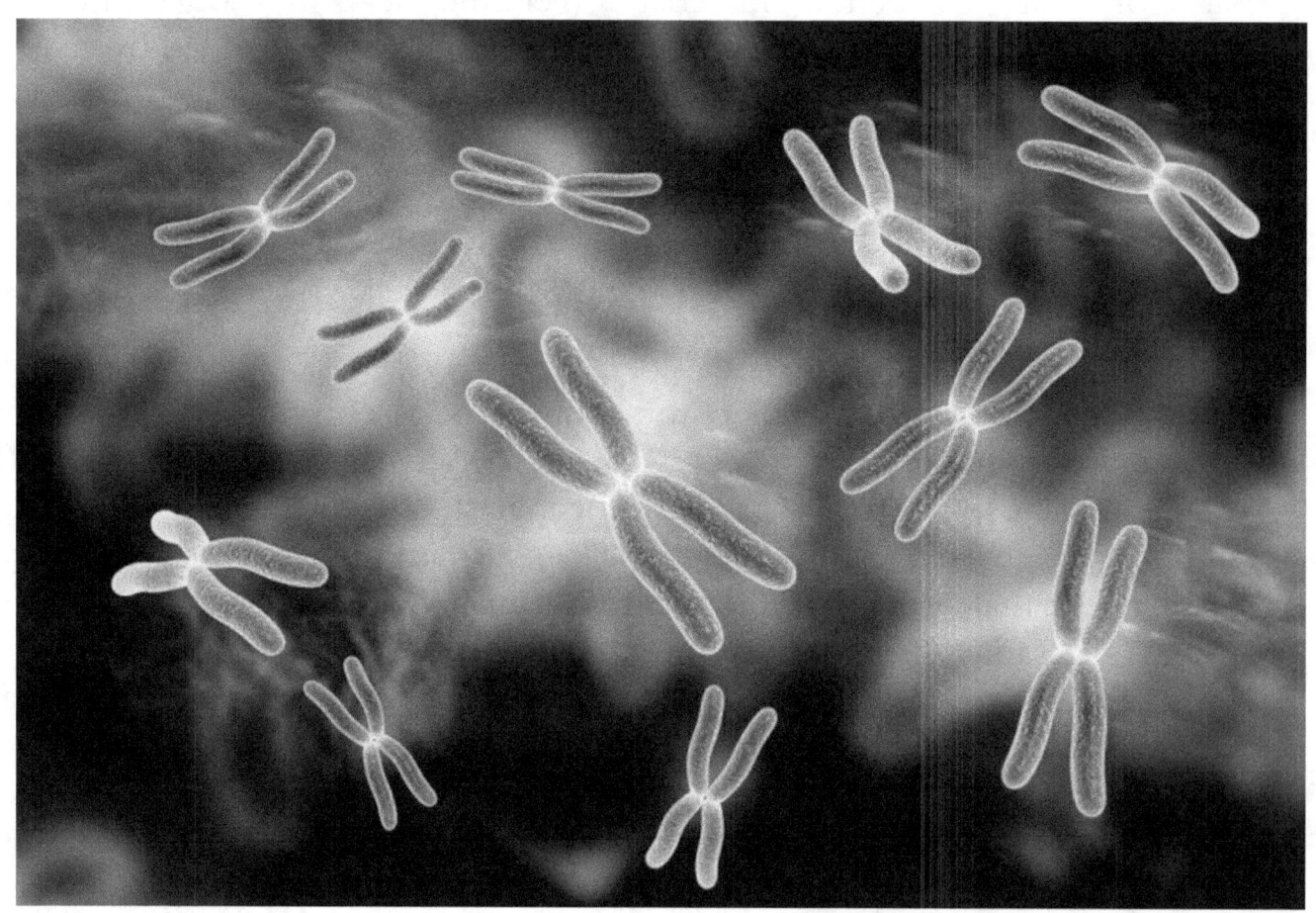

Chromosomes (microscope)

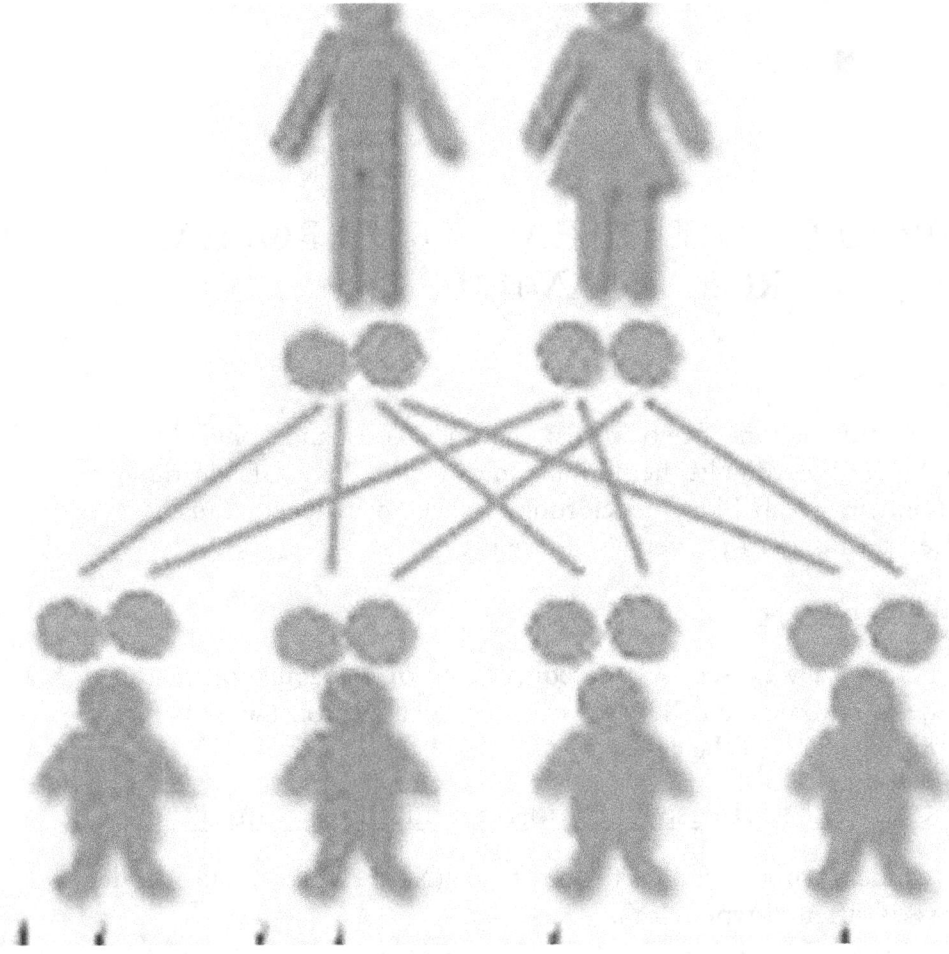

Transfer of Dominant Traits and Recessive Traits to the Offspring

HEMOPHILIA: THE DISEASE OF EUROPEAN ROYAL FAMILIES

What is Hemophilia?

Hemophilia is a combination of two words: "hemo", blood and "philia" which is related to love. Accordingly, hemophilia means the love of bleeding, a medical condition in which blood to clotting is severely reduced, causing the sufferer to bleed profusely from even a slight injury.

What Causes the Disease?

The condition is typically caused by a hereditary lack of a coagulation factor, a defect in a gene in chromosome X. Most often the coagulation factor is factor VIII. That represents 85% of the cases.

The Female Carries the Disease Chromosome but does Contract it!

The female gender chromosome is one type (XX), while male gender chromosome is of different types (XY).

If we assume that a female carries a defective chromosome related to hemophilia. She would not acquire the illness since there is another chromosome of the same type. The healthy chromosome compensates for the defective one. However, she can transfer the defective chromosome to her offsprings. The males will acquire hemophilia while the females will carry the disease without contracting it.

The odds of inheriting the defective chromosome is 50%; that is it is not necessarily that all her sons will acquire hemophilia.

Queen Victoria Spreads Hemophilia

The most famous hemophilia case in history and most well-known case of genetic diseases in general is the transfer of hemophilia from the British Queen Victoria (1819-1901) to three of her nine sons. Her son Prince Leopold acquired hemophilia while the disease was not transfer to his brother Prince Albert. Leopold did not live long as he died when he was 30 years old due to brain bleeding. Queen Victoria's daughters Alice and Beatrice carried the hemophilia chromosome. After their marriage and the marriage of the offsprings the hemophilia illness (defective chromosome) was spread among the European royal class; especially in Prussia (Germany now) Russia and Spain.

How Did Queen Victoria Acquire the Disease?

From where did Queen Victoria acquire the defective chromosome? There is no evidence that any of her ancestors had contracted the disease. It is also unlikely that she inherited the disease from her mother. Therefore, it is more likely that some type of gene mutation took place in the defective chromosome in Queen Victoria, which relates to the coagulation factor that reduces blood clotting.

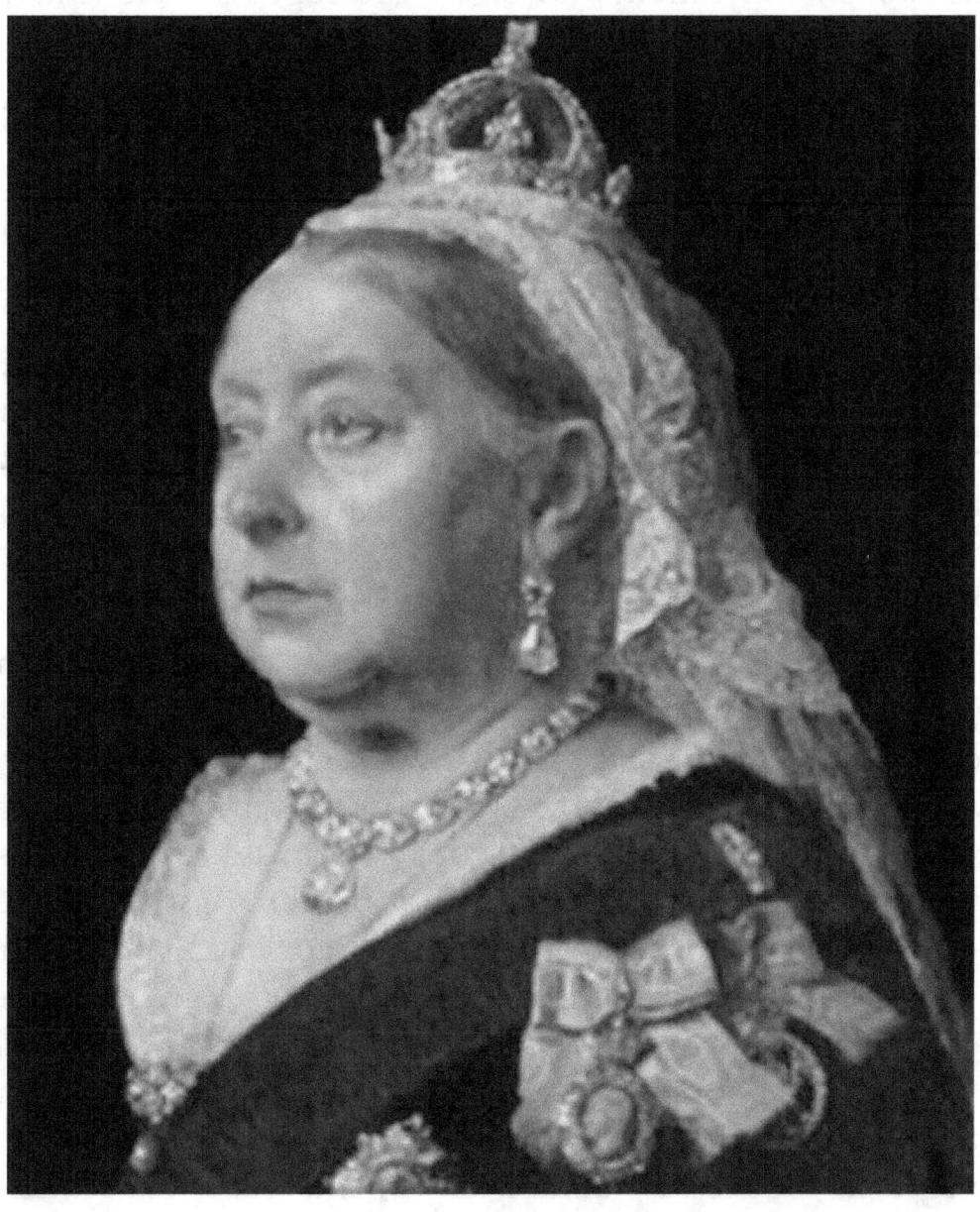

Queen Victoria

What are the Symptoms of Hemophilia?

The symptoms of acquiring hemophilia are exhibited in sudden continuous bleeding which may take place without any injury. The bleeding could be from the nose or in the urine. However, the most vulnerable organ to bleeding are the joints, especially the knee. The patient's knee would suddenly get swollen accompanied by excruciating pain that may hinder mobility. This is because of the accumulation of the blood in the joint's gaps. With the repetition of the bleeding the joint can be deteriorated. The body reacts to the bleeding by producing enzymes to digest that blood. While the bleeding may stop the enzymes action will continue to digest the edges of ligaments and may attack the joint's bone leading to deterioration and impacting the function of the joint.

This development reminds of a young man who used to come to my clinic. He was limping. He tries to lift his affected knee by hand to continue his walk.

Rasputin Treats the Son of the Tsar of Russia from Hemophilia!

Among the victims of hemophilia is Alexei Nikolaevich the last Tsesarevich and the heir to the Russian throne. He was the youngest child and only son of Emperor Nicholas II and Empress Alexandra Feodorovna. The disease was genetically transmitted to Alexei through marriage between Queen Victoria's daughters and European Princes. The Tsar himself was a cousin of the British King at that time.

During the summer of 1912, Alexei developed a hemorrhage in his thigh and groin after a jolting carriage ride near the royal hunting grounds, which caused a large hematoma. Alexandra, Alexei's mother sought the help of the family's close friend and confidant, the mystic and self-proclaimed holy man, Grigori Rasputin to treat her son through spiritual healing. As a self-proclaimed holy man who was regarded as a monk or pilgrim, Rasputin gained considerable influence in late imperial Russia. Alexandra appealed to Rasputin (who was in Siberia), asking him to pray for Alexei. Rasputin wrote back quickly, telling the tsarina that "God has seen your tears and heard your prayers. Do not grieve. The Little One will not die. Do not allow the doctors to bother him too much." The next morning, Alexei's condition was unchanged, but Alexandra was encouraged by the message and regained some hope that Alexei would survive. Alexei's bleeding stopped the following day.

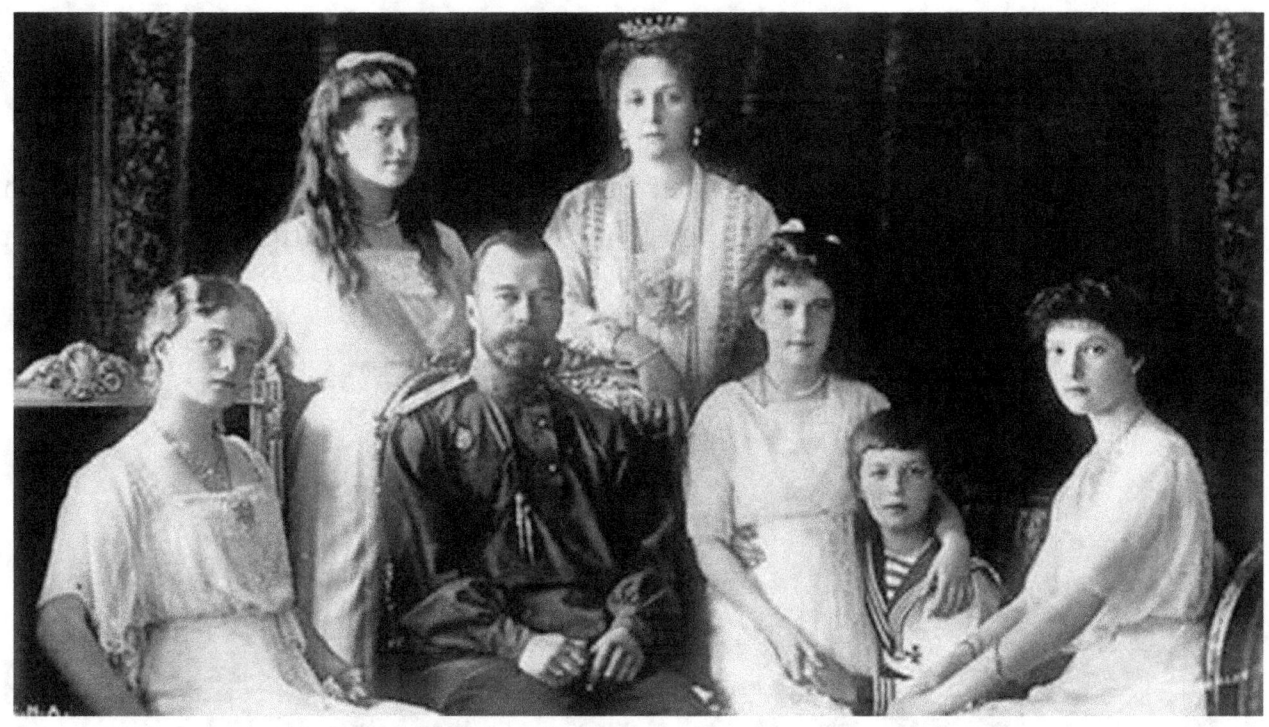

Nicholas II the Tsar of Russia with his family, he was executed by gunfire at the onset of the Bolshevik Revolution in 1917.

Alexei's recovery "one of the most mysterious episodes of the whole Rasputin legend". The cause of his recovery is unclear: Massie speculated that Rasputin's suggestion not to let doctors disturb Alexei had aided his recovery by allowing him to rest and heal, or that his message may have aided Alexei's recovery by calming Alexandra and reducing the emotional stress on Alexei. Alexandra, however, believed that Rasputin had performed a miracle, and concluded that he was essential to Alexei's survival. Some claim that Rasputin stopped Alexei's bleeding on other occasions through hypnosis.

Rasputin gained himself the title of "false prophet and even an Antichrist" as he was accused of religious heresy and rape, was suspected of exerting undue political influence over the tsar, and was even rumored to be having an affair with the tsarina. the local clergy denounced Rasputin as a heretic. Rumors were spread and multiplied that Rasputin had assaulted female followers and behaved inappropriately on visits to the royal family – and particularly with the Tsar's teenage daughters Olga and Tatyana.

Is there a treatment for Hemophilia?

The only available treatment for hemophilia is the injection of the patient with clotting agents, which can be prepared from donated blood. The treatment is effective in stopping the bleeding. In that case the patient should not take in blood thinning drugs such as aspirin.

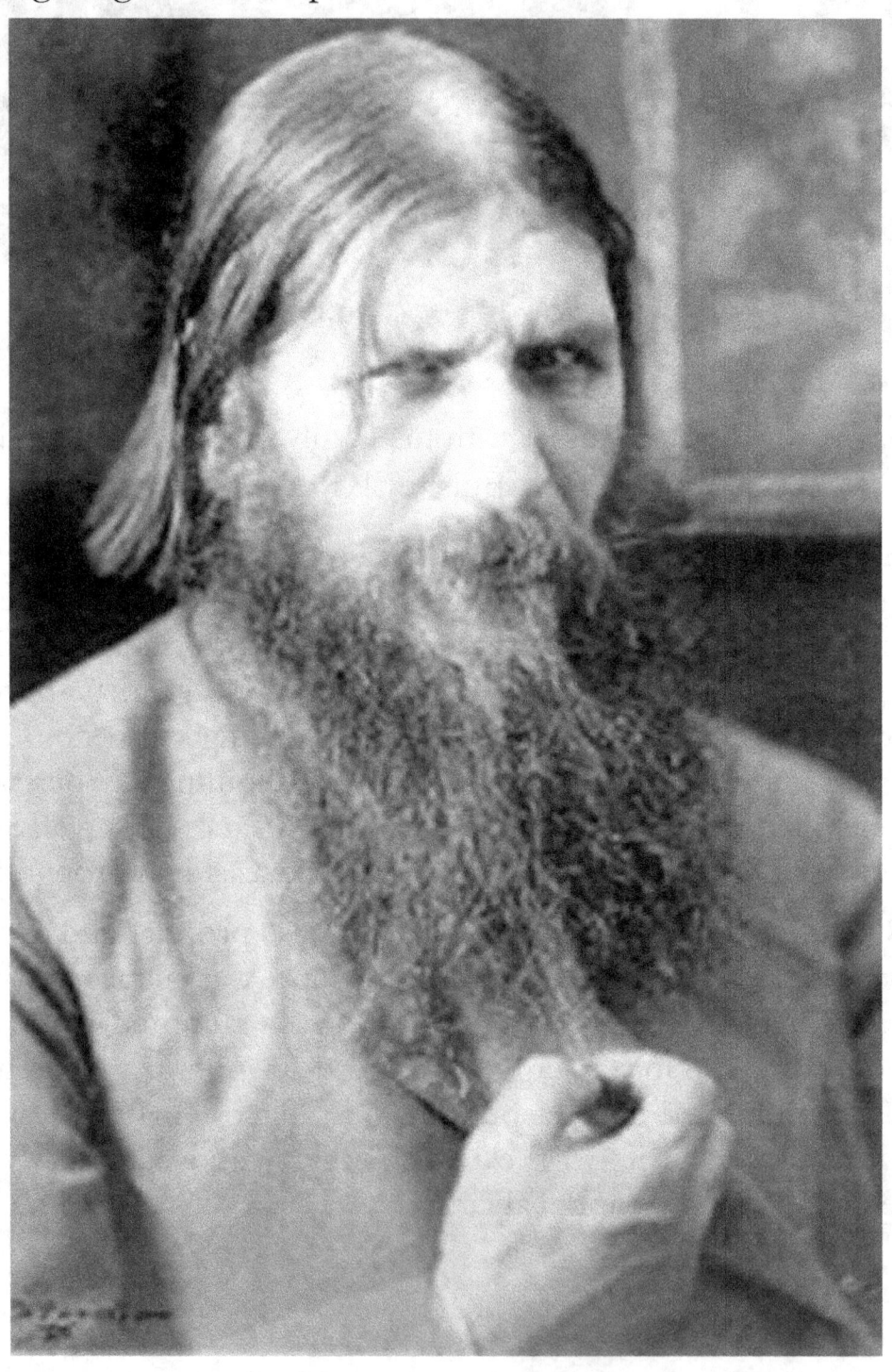

What is the Extent of the Spread of Hemophilia?

Hemophilia cases are limited. During my practice as a physician I knew only of three families in Alexandria wherein members of the family had hemophilia. They were known to all physicians in town by name.

Prevention

It is possible to identify the defective gene that causes hemophilia before marriage, and during pregnancy to take preventive measures to avoid having offsprings suffering from hemophilia.

HERE IS AMERICA: ARE YOU WHITE, BLACK OR RED

If You Are Black …

Blacks from African origin are less lucky than white American, since they are more susceptible to contracting dangerous diseases, such as sickle cell anemia, diabetes mellitus, pancreatic cancer and COVID-19.

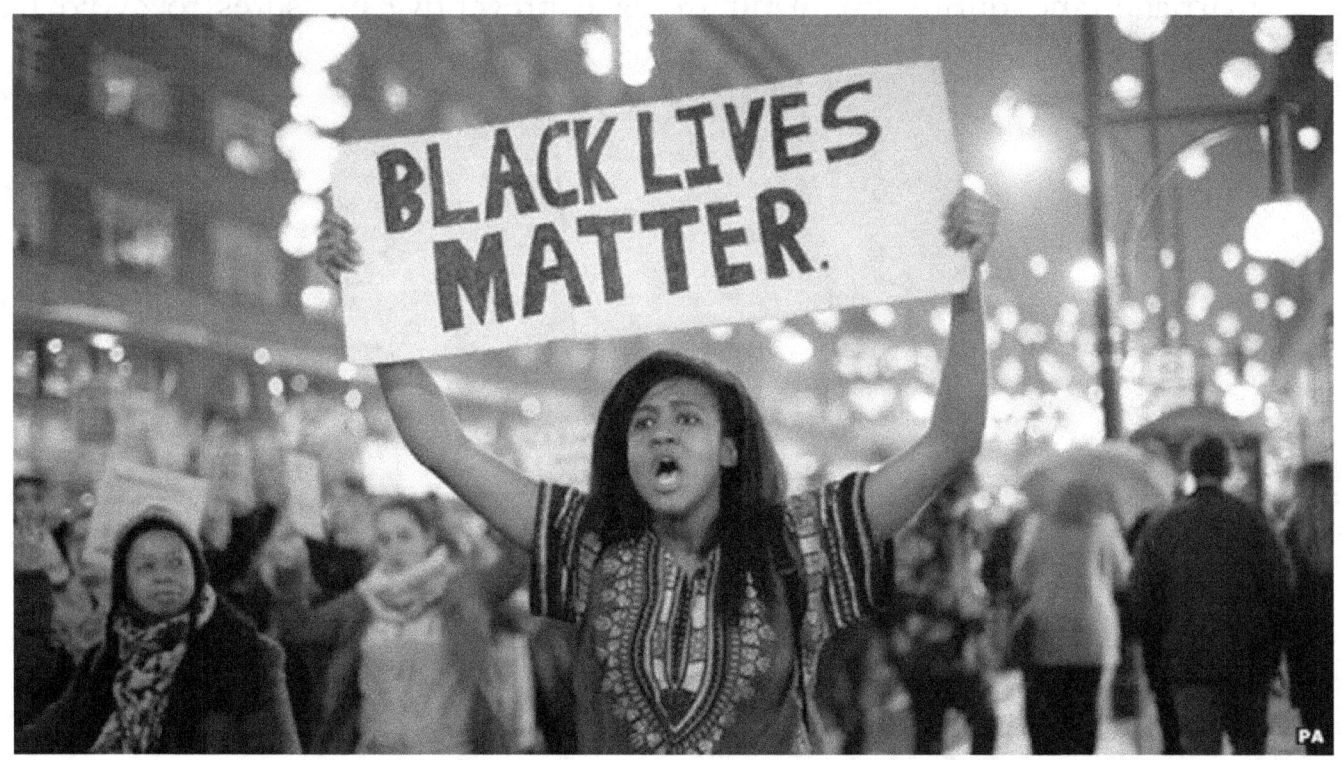

Black community

If You Are White …

White people, with the great differences between their ancestry, are generally susceptible to skin cancer compared to those with black or dark skin. However, why is that?

The light tender skin has a small ration of melanin. Those cells are responsible for the color of the skin. This is while black people have a large percentage of melanin which turns their skin dark. Such color differential is associated with the genes.

Why does the Complexions Darken When Exposed to Sunrays?

Darkening of the bare skin as it is exposed to the sunrays for an elongated period of time works to our advantage, in realty. That results from the concentration of melanin in those exposed areas of our body to protect the skin from the harmful effects of sunrays. The most pronounced harmful effect is the development of skin cancerous cells.

If You are Red…

The red here is intended to reference the Native American race which is often called the Red Indians. They represent 1.5% of the population in the USA. They earned that name because when Columbus reached the shores of the West Indies, he thought that he had arrived at India so he called the natives Indians. Later the adjective Red was added to distinguish between them and the inhabitants of India. In realty their complexions have a trace of red color.

Some of the Red Indians assimilated with the community and others preferred to live in the reservations and maintain their ancestors' lifestyle.

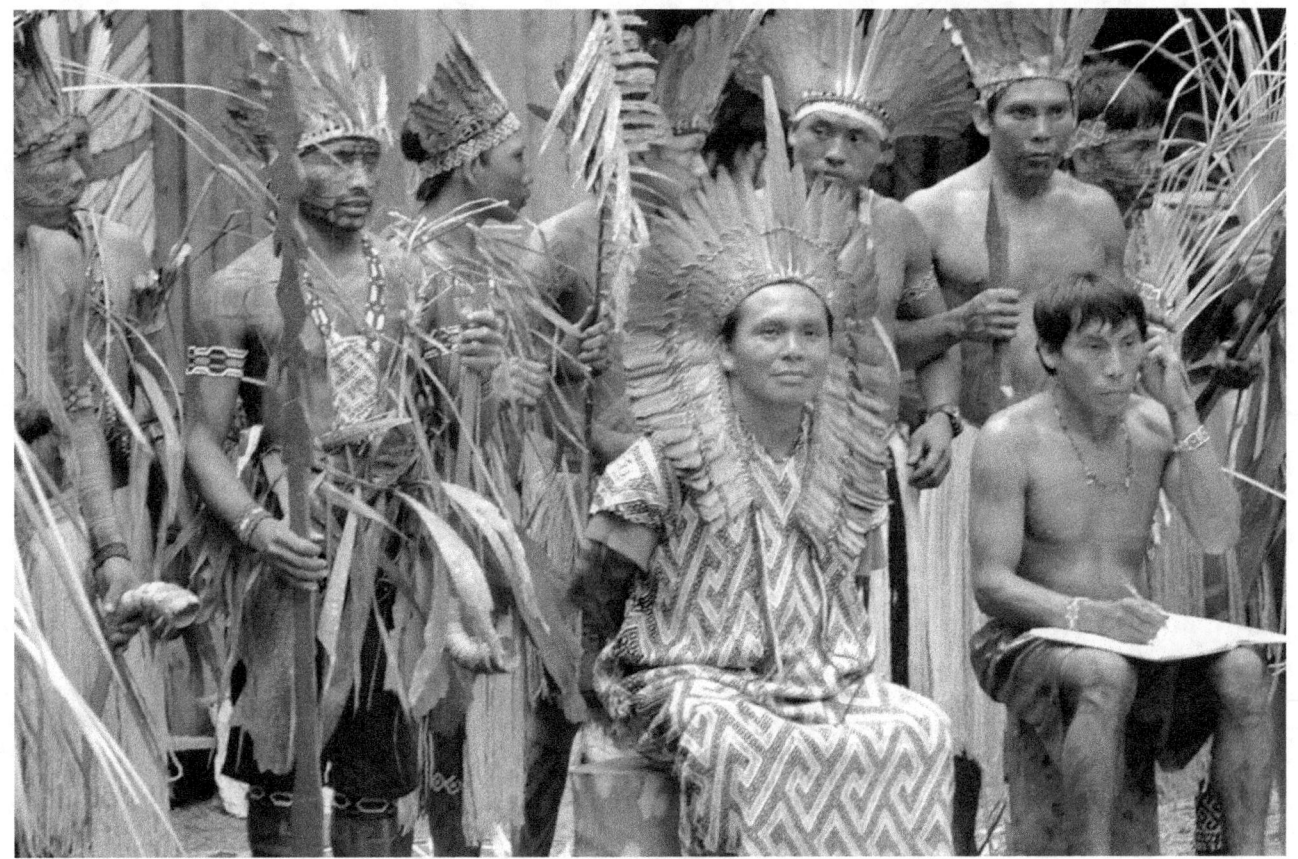

Red Indians Tribe

Diabetes

It seems that the Red Indian race have inherited the diabetes disease since the ratio of those who have diabetes is around 40% of their population. This is the highest ratio of diabetes among the different and distinctive races comprising the US population. Most of the diabetes cases involving Native Americans are type 2. This is especially the case among those who assimilated into the common American lifestyle, followed the common diet that lead to increase in weight and subsequent increase in resistance of insulin effectiveness. In fact the percentage of those who have diabetes among Native Americans is higher than the corresponding ratio among African Americans.

Wrinkles

It seems that the Native Americans are more susceptible than other races to develop wrinkles at a relatively young age and add to their faces a stern look. This maybe attributed to their genetic makeup.

WHAT IS SICKLE CELL ANEMIA?

In the USA, the sickle cell anemia is limited to African Americans. However, outside the USA the disease is found among other races, as is the case in Asia, especially India.

Red blood cells are naturally round as the name indicates; however, in the presence of sickle cell anemia, the shape of the red blood cell is sickle-shaped or like a crescent.

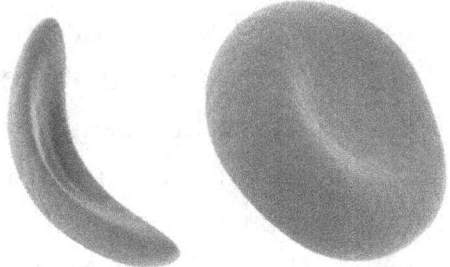

Red blood cell normal (round) and sickle-shaped

The abnormal red blood cells are associated with a defect in the hereditary gene responsible for the formation of hemoglobin which results in deformation of the shape of the crier red blood cells which transfer oxygen to the body cells. Such gene is recessive and is inherited from the parents.

What is the Harm from the Distorted Shape of the Red Blood Cells?

The harm from the distorted shape of the red blood cells can be seen from the behavior of the sickle cells:

- Difficulty in flowing through the blood vessels,
- Not flexible,
- Ease of being obstructed in a narrow blood vessel,
- Can be fractured through the trip across blood vessels,
- Lower carrying capacity of oxygen (hemoglobin),
- May cause obstruction of blood vessels, which results in depriving an organ from the required amount of oxygen.

This is in addition to the fact that the deformed red blood cells have a life expectancy of between 10 to 20 days which is much lower than the life expectancy of normal red blood cells which reaches 120 days.

How Does the Patient Feel?

As any type of anemia, the patient gets tired from minimal physical activity, pale, slow in growth, comprised immunity system and can be easily and repeatedly infected by pneumonia or the common cold. This is in addition to exposure to more serious complications as a result of the erratic movement of the blood flow as well as clogging of the blood vessels, for example:

- Deterioration of the internal organs such as the heart, liver and spline.
- The spline is especially affected since its function is the purification of the blood from broken and defective cells. The presence of sickle cells increases the load on the spline as a result of the accumulation of blood in the relatively narrow blood cells and subsequent deterioration of the tissue of the spline in a way that make it vulnerable to any infection.
- Susceptibility to strokes as a result of irregular blood flow and the increased likelihood of blood clotting.
- Problems in the heart because of irregular blood flow.
- Jaundice as a result of broken red blood cells and the seepage of the hemoglobin in the blood and its conversion to bilirubin; a yellow substance that results in yellowing the color of the skin and the sclera (the white of the eye) and results also in a brownish or dark yellow urine.
- Formation of stones in the gallbladder as a result of the increase in bilirubin.
- Ulcers in the leg due to constriction in blood vessels.
- Erectile disfunction due to the slow flow of blood in the penis.
- Complications in the eyesight leading to blindness due to constriction of blood flow in the cornea.
- Pulmonary hypertension and hard breathing.
- Death.

Those Cannot Fly!

As we move to high altitude, there is less oxygen in the air that you breathe. This means that all the blood from all areas of the lungs, is relatively short on oxygen or hypoxic. This happens if we move to high mountains or fly. This causes complications to those suffering from sickle cell diseases who suffer from lower oxygen in their blood.

How Can I Tell if My Child is Suffering from Sickle Cell Anemia?

Sickle cell anemia is a hereditary disease that is transferred to the offsprings and appears on children upon birth.

The disease can be diagnosed by testing the blood, especially the hemoglobin. The hemoglobin can be separated by electrophoresis and detect abnormal hemoglobin.

Is there a Cure for Sickle Cell Anemia?

As any other hereditary disease, there is no treatment for the disease or any drugs to eliminate it. However, bone marrow transplant can be used to produce healthy red blood cells. Such procedure yields successful results, especially with children. To control the progress of the disease and its complications, some medications may be administered to enhance blood flow and prevent the blood cells damage.

AMERICA RANKS FIRST IN DIABETES

Statistics

According to the British Daily Mail, the USA ranks first in the World in terms of the number of cases of diabetes which reaches 30 million. Most of the cases are Type 2 Diabetes.

What is the Difference between Type 1 and Type 2 Diabetes?

In Type 1 Diabetes the pancreas produces insufficient insulin or no insulin at all and accordingly injection of insulin is necessary.

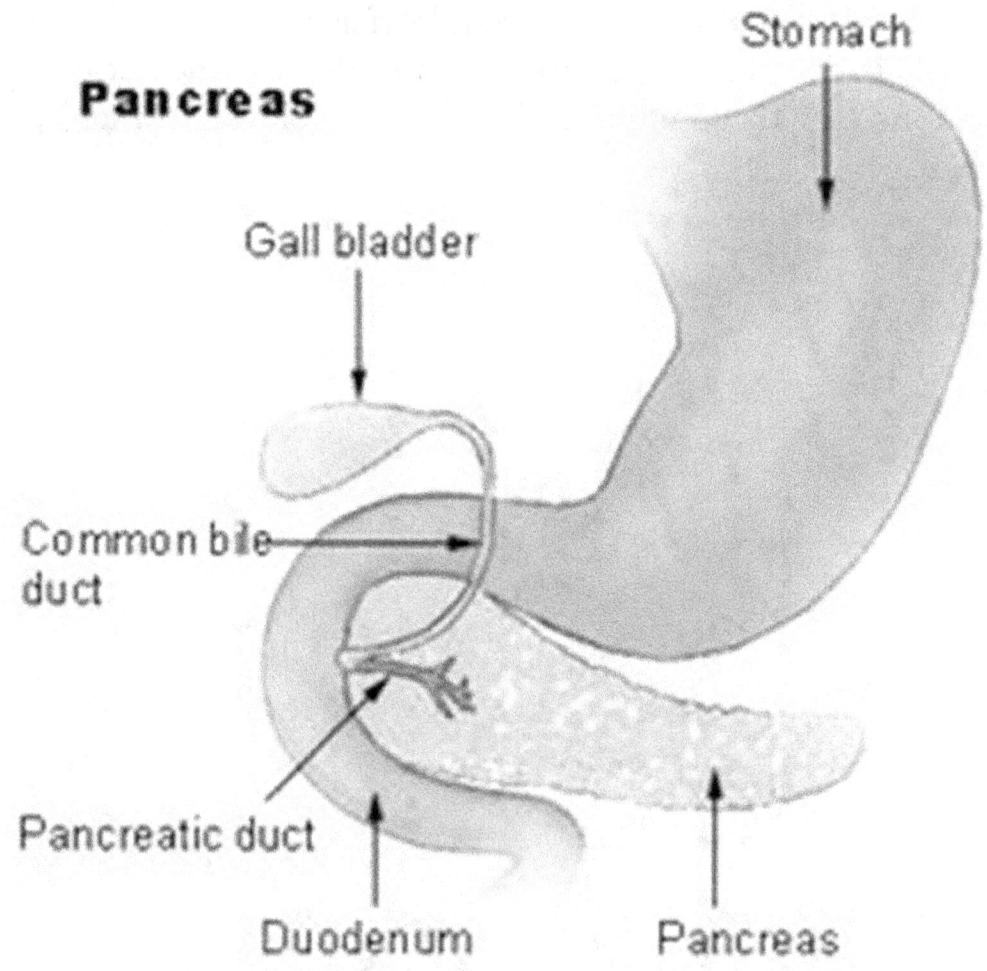

The pancreas participates in the process of food digestion through the beta cells that produces insulin

Type 1 Diabetes is a chronic condition that starts early in life (the childhood or adolescence) and the patient suffers from complications that are not present in Type 2 diabetes.

However, what are the causes?

There are no clear causes, however, it is known is that the immune system — which normally fights harmful bacteria or viruses — attacks the beta cells (β cells) (insulin-producing cells in the pancreas) and destroys them by mistake. This leaves the patient with little or no insulin. Instead of being transported into your cells, sugar builds up in your bloodstream. Beta cells make up 50–70% of the cells in human islets. In patients with type I or type II diabetes, beta-cell mass and function are diminished, leading to insufficient insulin secretion and hyperglycemia. Beta cells may be destroyed also by a virus.

Type 1 is thought to be caused by a combination of genetic susceptibility and environmental factors, though exactly what those factors are is still unclear. Weight is not believed to be a factor in type 1 diabetes.

Genetic susceptibility is connected to a defect in the KCNJ11 gene that controls the production of insulin. The KCNJ11 (Potassium Inwardly Rectifying Channel Subfamily J Member 11) is a Protein Coding gene. Diseases associated with KCNJ11 include Hyperinsulinemic Hypoglycemia, Familial, 2 and Maturity-Onset Diabetes of The Young, Type 13.

The pancreas in Type 2 diabetes is capable of producing insulin, nevertheless the produced insulin may be limited or not enough to be effective enough as needed. This is why this type of diabetes can be treated by drug regulating the blood sugar (glucose). This type appears at a relatively older age (forties).

Weight is a factor in type 2 diabetes. There is a connection between the prevalence of the disease and obesity as well as unhealthy diets. Accordingly, the disease can be controlled by the proper diet. Other factors include psychological stress.

Is Diabetes Hereditary?

It is amazing that hereditary diabetes is more prevalent in the type 2 than type 1. If either parents or any of family member suffers from type 2, there is a chance that a family member will get type 2 diabetes. The symptoms may be triggered by continuous or repeated psychological stresses.

Acquisition of the diabetes is dependent on the race as it is higher among African black Americans (more than 13%) than among white Americans (about 8.7%).

In a study by the American Medical Society showed that the percentage of black women with diabetes is more than three times than white women suffering from diabetes.

Most of the cases are Type 2 diabetes.

Barbershop and Analysis Lab!

It is amazing that the black barbershops in the USA offers the services of testing the sugar level. This is of great importance since it contributes to early discovery of the disease which may have no clear symptoms at the onset.

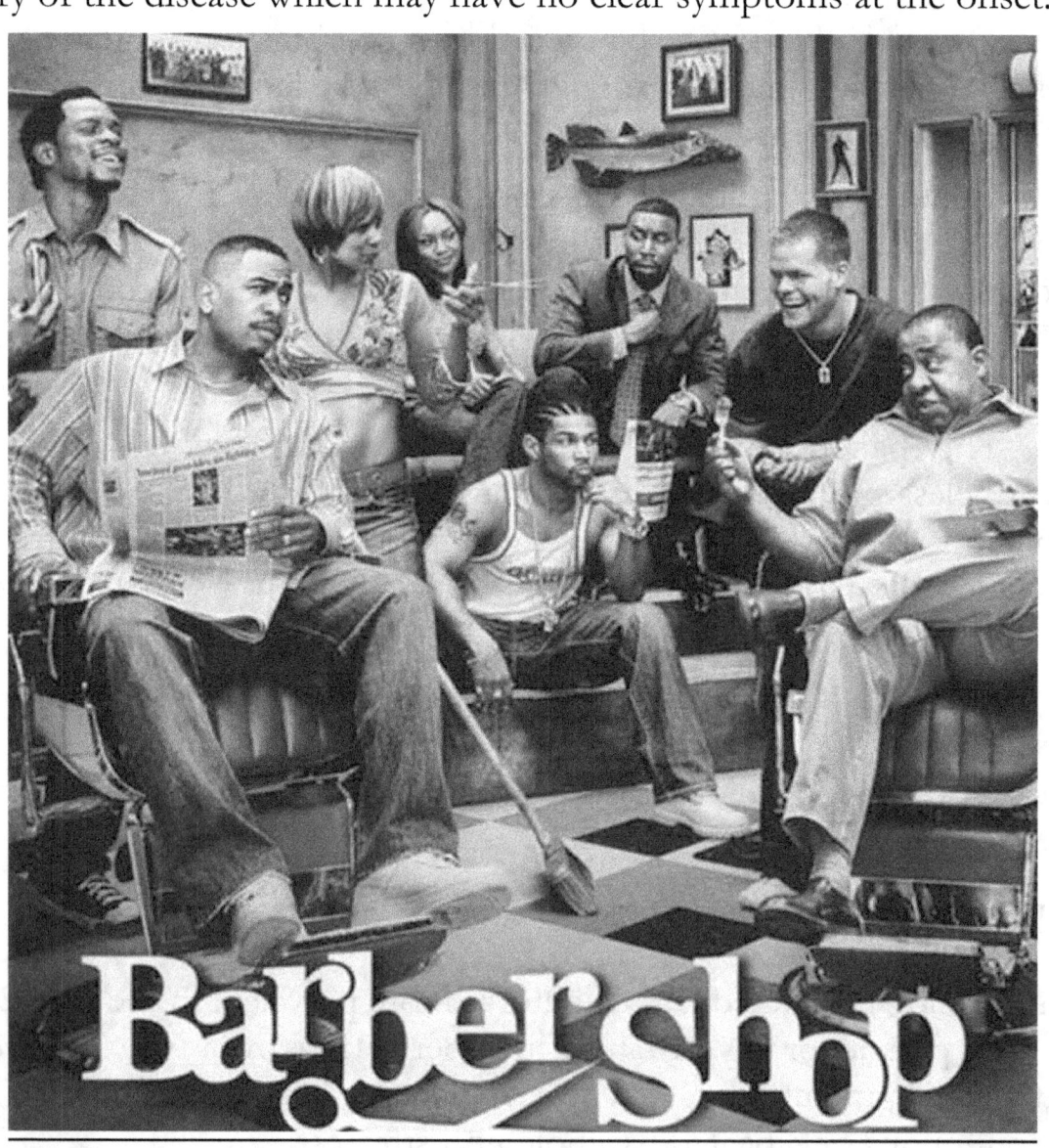

It is also amazing that such barbershops are a manifestation of social clubs and country clubs in the white community. Customers of the barbershops exchange conversations and complaints which releases some of the tension in place of rushing to psychiatrists and psychologists seeking treatment!

Warnings that Should not be Ignored …

In quiet a few cases, diabetes is discovered by mere accident through routine blood work. In other cases, there are symptoms that could be a prewarning of diabetes. Such symptoms must not be ignored. Those include:

- Frequent urination: this is a way of ridding the body from excess blood sugar.
- Dry mouth: results from frequent urination.
- Fatigue: This occurs despite congestion of a sufficient nutritional foods and is a result of the inability to convert blood sugar into energy for the cells.
- Vaginal itching: inflammation accompanied with itching due to yeast infection.

PANCREATIC CANCER AT A HIGH PERCENTAGE AMONG BLACK AMERICANS

Studies

Pancreatic cancer was the subject of studies performed in Atlanta, Detroit and New Jersey for about three years from 1986 to 1989. The studies revealed that the percentage of infected by pancreatic cancer among African Americans exceeds from 23% to 52% among white Americans.

Causes

The pancreatic cancer studies concurred on some factors that contribute to the contraction of the disease; most of which are prevalent among black people in general. Those are:

- Race: The disease is prevailing among the black race. In some black families the percentage is as high as 46% compared to 37% among white families. The studies have not revealed a defective gene that causes acquisition of the disease.
- Diabetes: A factor that is more prevalent among blacks.
- Weight: Increase in BMI (Body Mass Index= wight/height). Obesity is more prevalent among blacks; especially women, compared to white women.
- Smoking: Another important factor which is more prevalent among blacks.
- Pancreatitis: Pancreas inflammation (pancreatitis) may be acute or chronic. Blacks are more vulnerable to chronic pancreatitis which increases the chances for pancreatic cancer.
- Alcohol: Drinking alcohol increases the chance of acquiring pancreatic cancer; especially in case of addiction or excess.
- Socioeconomic Conditions: The socioeconomical differential between blacks and whites is staggering. In some cases, addiction of alcohol and smoking is tied to the quality of life.
- Black Women are more Susceptible to Pancreatic Cancer: Excessive or moderate alcohol drinking in addition to high BMI among black women increases their vulnerability to pancreatic cancer by about 88% while the combination of obesity and addiction among white women increases their

susceptibility to the disease to 47% only. If both factors disappeared among black and white women, the chances of contracting pancreatic cancer levels out to be almost the same.

- ❖ High Consumption of Processed Meat: Excess in consumption of processed fatty meats such as ham and bacon that contains nitrates enhances the chances of pancreatic cancer as well as cancer in general.

Late Diagnosis

Statistics have shown that most pancreatic cancer cases among blacks are diagnosed at a later stage which is incurable in contrast the diagnosis of the disease among whites. This may be connected to the lack of healthcare for blacks.

Where is the Pancreas and what its Function?

The pancreas is located behind the stomach. It secretes pancreatic bile (for digestion) and its beta cells produce insulin to burn the sugar in the blood (glucose).

Due to the back location of the pancreas, it is difficult to examine it by ultrasonic or sound imaging of the stomach. Furthermore, some of the pancreatic problems can be confused with stomach upset or indigestion and inflammation of the gallbladder. Accordingly, detection of problems associated with the pancreas may be delayed or neglected.

The pancreas comprises: head, neck, body and tail. The tail looks like the tip of the tongue. The head is on the other side of the tail.

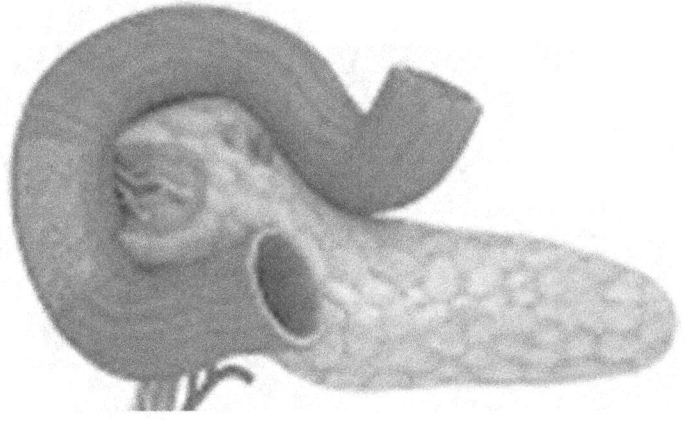

Tumor of the Head of the Pancreas

Expected Symptoms of Pancreatic Cancer

In many cases the symptoms or the early signs are hard to identify and may not clearly show, however with the growth of the cancer tumor, the symptoms and complications start to be obvious:

- Pain at the top of the belly with echo in the back.
- Weight loss.
- Loss of appetite.
- Lethargy and fatigue.
- Diabetes or the loss of control on the diabetes if it is already there.
- Paleness takes place when the tumor of the pancreatic head blocks the flow of the bile through the common bile duct. In this case the color of the skin turns yellowish, the urine become dark, the fesses color fades away and the skin started to itch.

Treatment

The treatment depends on the stage of the tumor growth. The tumor may be removed or the physician may advise of chemotherapy.

CORONAVIRUS SPREAD AMONG BLACKS

In the USA, where I currently reside, the number of blacks who fell victims of COVID-19 much exceeds the number of whites. According to one of the statistical sources the percentage of blacks who tested positive is about 70%.

Is that related to race?

The answer is yes. It is true but we have to also consider other factors leading to such out of proportion increase; compared to the white, such as:

- Poverty and the decline of the living standard of a large percentage of blacks.
- The crowded housing resulting from unaffordable housing for the poor.
- Poor health care.
- The spread of chronic diseases among blacks, especially diabetes.

Potential Coronavirus Symptoms

There is a flood of information about COVID-19 which we have been facing for quite a while until now. Such information is evolving continuously. At the onset of the pandemic in the USA the CDC indicated that 20% of the coronavirus cases do not exhibit any clear symptoms …

Yet a study in Ochsner hospital showed that 75% of the cases do not exhibit any clear symptoms!

Nevertheless, the possible symptoms of the infection did not change much. Those are such as: rise in body temperature, headache, sore throat, dry persistent cough, runny nose, loss of ability to taste and effect on the olfactory senses, possible diarrhea, nausia and vomiting, and hard breathing at an advanced stage.

FACTORS PROMOTING SKIN CANCER

Skin cancer is one of the cancers that is widely spread in the USA as well as all around the world. Statistically about a million American are diagnosed yearly of having skin cancer.

The most prominent factor leading to this type of cancer is the extensive exposure to the sunrays and more specifically to ultraviolet (UV) radiation which comprises two types A and B. Most likely, UVB is the type which is responsible for skin cancer since it leads to causing damage to the DNA in a manner that it changes the normal cell and turn it into cancerous cells that grow in an uncontrolled abnormal fashion.

The Left Side of the Body is the Most Vulnerable!

It is quite interesting to notice that the skin cancer is more inclined to attack the left side of the body, such as the face and the arm. Such observation is evident in those who drive long distances in the sun wherein their left side is exposed to direct sun rays compared to their righthand side.

Do You Have a Nevus on Your Body?

The nevus is a birthmark or a mole on the skin, especially a birthmark in the form of a raised red patch. It is basically a mass of melanin cells that appears as a raised brown or a black lump. Whether it is a beauty mark, mole, nevus or birthmark it is a skin pigmented skin lesion.

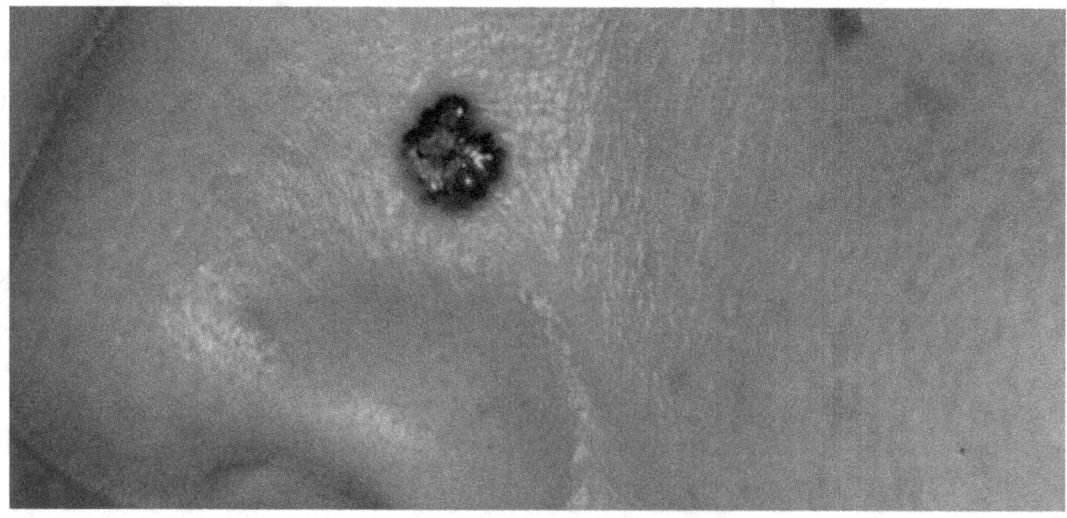

Malignant nevus

By exposure to sunrays, the nevus can be easily changed to a melanin cancerous tumor known as Melanoma. This is one of the most dangerous types of skin cancer. There are an estimated 200 thousand cases of Melanoma yearly in the USA; most of them are white.

Signs that Must not be Ignored ...

It is necessary to consult with a specialist physician if any change occurred to a nevus, which was preset for long time; when:

- Change in color,
- Increase in size,
- Hemorrhage,
- Appearance of surface corrugation,
- Irregular growth on the sides.

This is in addition to the awareness of a Positive Family History; that is a member of the family has suffered from skin cancer. This is because the hereditary melanin could have been deformed. This leads to formation of skin cancer due to deformation in the gene POT1 which provides the protection. This gene is transferred to offsprings.

Beware of Sunbathing by the Seashore!

Sunbathing by the seashore with the objective of tanning is a popular sport, especially among women. However, such sunbathing poses great harm to the skin especially if it reached burning the skin, a big factor in developing skin cancer.

Excessive Smoking

Excessive smoking could play a role in susceptibility to skin cancer in the facial locations exposed to heavy smoking. This is especially dangerous if combined to intensive exposure to sunrays or the presence of nevi.

Use of Drugs to Weaken Immunity

There are drugs administered to weaken the Immunity system to treat autoimmune diseases such as the Systemic Lupus erythematosus (SLE). Those drugs and especially Azathioprine can promote the formation of skin cancerous cells. Furthermore, skin cancer may easily take place in cases wherein the Immunity system such as the case of AIDS patients.

Is There a Benefit in Using Sun Protection Aids?

Yes, Sunscreen reflects or absorbs UV in a way that can minimize the harm it may cause and reduces the chances of development of skin cancer. It also protects from early development of wrinkles.

There is an ongoing debate regarding the safety of using such formulations on the complexions, nevertheless there is no proof that they will cause and harm.

WHY AMERICANS ARE MORE SUSCEPTIBLE TO DIVERTICULOSIS?

The Disease Connected Generally to Americans!

Throughout my work as a physician specialized in internal medicine in the Middle East, I came across a myriad of colon diseases. Nevertheless, I have never encountered on case of diverticulosis. However, when I visited the USA, I noticed the wide spread of the disease among all Americans from different races, while the percentage is higher among whites. This is understood since most Americans are white. Diverticulosis is also found in Europe but with lower percentage of the population. This is why diverticulosis is called the Western Disease.

In the USA the yearly victims of diverticulosis reach 200 thousand. Contracting the disease is usually for people after age 40. The risk of getting the disease increases after reaching 60 years of age.

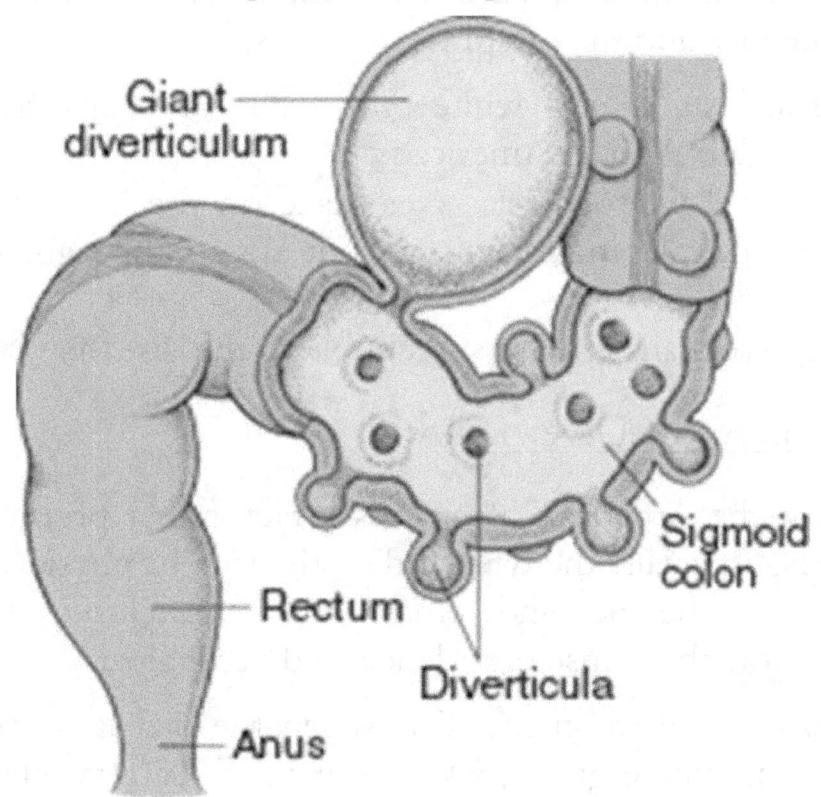

Diverticulosis

The diverticulosis disease takes different forms. It takes place when pockets (diverticula) form in the walls of the digestive tract. The inner layer of the intestine pushes through weak spots in the outer lining. This pressure makes them bulge out, making little pouches. Most often it happens in the colon, the lower part of your large intestine. The disease occurs at different levels. It may be limited to one pouch or more in the colon. Also, the pouches differ in size, small or large.

What is Meant by Diverticulosis?

Diverticulum is formed at a weak spot in the smooth muscles lining the colon, such as the entrance of a blood vessel. Such diverticula may be formed in different week locations in the colon. Accordingly, the disease is called diverticulosis. It is similar to the formation of hernia.

Is Diverticulosis Hereditary?

It is unlikely that the diverticulosis disease is hereditary. No abnormal gene related to the diverticulosis has been discovered. Nevertheless, the disease is more prevalent in some families than others. In addition, there are differences related to the race and the offsprings, such as:

- Diverticulosis affects white Americans at a slightly higher percentage compared to African Americans.
- Usually the diverticulosis takes place on the left side in Americans (the Western people, in general) while it affects the right side of people from Asian heritage.
- Asian Americans are less susceptible to the disease.

Potential Causes of Diverticulosis

It seems that the American lifestyle is a factor that promotes the presence of diverticulosis, especially the type of diet, the lack of physical activity and obesity caused by both the diet and lethargy. This conclusion is supported by the following factors that cause prevalence of diverticulosis:

- ❖ Shortage of fibers in the diet: When the diet lacks fibers, such as those present in whole grains, whole flour and leafy vegetables, the volume of waste (feces) shrinks. With the continuous lack of fibers, the diameter of the colon shrinks. This leads to increase in the pressure of the refuse on the colon walls (per LaPlace Law) and thus the promotion of weak tissues wherein the pockets develop.

- ❖ Excess in consumption of red meat: Red meat is a basic food in most American meals. It was found that there is a relationship between excess in red meat consumption and diverticulosis. This is why vegetarians hardly suffer from diverticulosis.
- ❖ Negligence of physical activities: The decrease in physical activities lengthen the transit time of body waste in the colon before it leaves the body. Accordingly, the pressure increases on the walls of the colon. This causes weakness in some locations in the colon leading to the formation of one pocket or more.
- ❖ Constipation: Constipation leads to the buildup of pressure on the walls of the colon. In turn, this causes weakness in some locations in the colon leading to the formation of one pocket or more.
- ❖ Obesity: The chances of diverticulosis are enhanced by increase in the body mass.
- ❖ Some medications: Administration of some medications over a long period of time or repeatedly increases the chance of diverticulosis. Among such medicine antiinflammation non-cortisone medications (NSAIDs) which are used to alleviate joint pain.
- ❖ Marfan Syndrome: People suffering from the Marfan Syndrome are likely to develop diverticulosis.

However, what is the Marfan Syndrome?

Marfan syndrome (MFS) is a genetic disorder that affects the connective tissue. The connective tissues support and anchor body organs and other structures in the body, including the colon.

A person with MFS suffers from weakness in the connective tissues as a result of change in the FBN1 gene. Such defective genes transfers by heredity. weakness of the connective tissues that support and anchor the digestive system increases the chance for diverticulosis. This is why diverticulosis is hereditary in this case; however, the diverticulosis is associated with other problems such as elongation of Aortic Aneurysm.

Those with the MFS tend to be tall and thin, with long arms, legs, fingers and toes. They also typically have overly flexible joints and scoliosis. The overly flexibility is caused by weakness in the connective tissues of the joints and muscles.

I still recall the first case of MFS I have witnessed during my studies in the Medical School. The person with MFS was able to bend one of his hand fingers backward at very wide angle due to their flexibility. That was a great surprise to the students. However, such cases are rare. Those with MFS appear in movies and shows to display their amazing flexibility. This is in addition to being tall to a degree that attracts the attention!

President Abraham Lincoln is the most famous person with Marfan syndrome.

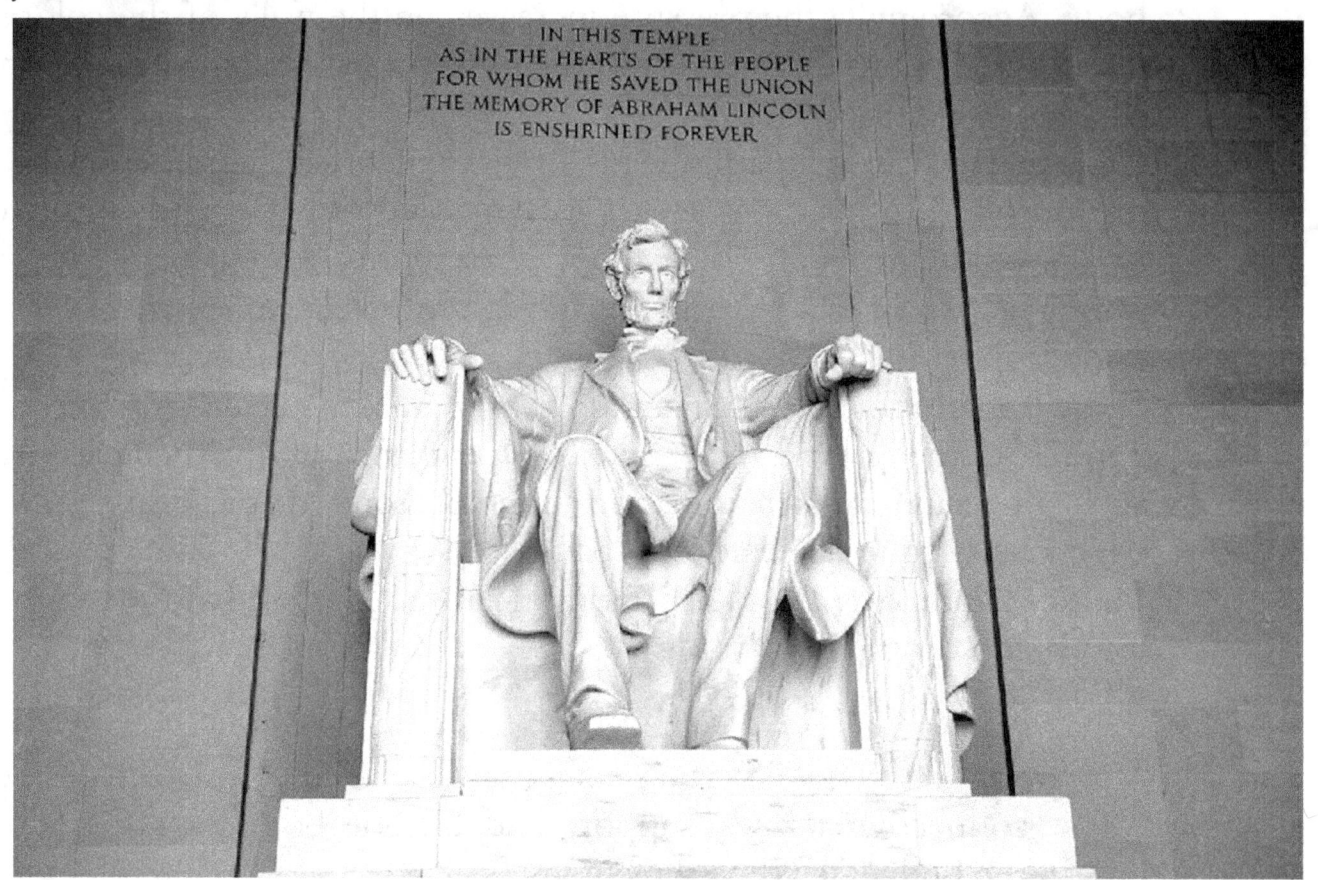

President Abraham Lincoln

What are the Symptoms of Diverticulosis?

The diverticulitis may stay dormant until the inflammation of one of the pockets. Symptoms such as those of nervous colon and abdominal bloating may take place. Passing gas is unusually loud because of trapping the gas in the pockets.

Accordingly, the actual percent of the spread of diverticulitis cannot be exactly determined. As long as there are no symptoms or difficulties the presence of diverticulitis does not come to attention and can go on without treatment.

What Causes Pocket Inflammation?

Diverticulitis is not a simple disease. On the contrary it could become very serious because of severe complications.

The accumulation of body waste in the formed pockets could lead to infection as any accumulation of any matter in the body. This infection could result from the bacteria associated with the feces. It is also possible that the wall of the pocket, which is already weak can be inflamed due to the increasing pressure of the waste and plugging of the pocket.

Such complications do not take place for all diverticulitis patients. However, they are likely to occur with advance in age. 10% of diverticulitis patients may suffer from inflammation of the pockets after the age of 40. However, after the age of 60 years the percentage can go as high as 50%. This increase is caused by the same factors that enhance contracting diverticulitis in the first place, such as lack of fibers, excessive red meat consumption, lack of physical activities and administration of anti-inflammation, non-cortisone medication, such as ibuprofen. It was also found that deficiency in vitamin D, which is often due to avoiding exposure to the sun increases the chances of inflammation of the colon pockets and the intestines in general.

Symptoms

Inflammation of colon pockets can be acute with severe symptoms or could be chronic with less severe and repetitive symptoms. The symptoms include:
- abdominal pain,
- tenderness and tension in the stomach,
- fever,
- nausea,
- light red blood in the stool, and
- a change in bowel habits: constipation with rare diarrhea.

Complications

Colonic perforation may take place in the inflamed pocket causing infection. An abscess may be formed and clogging of the intestines. Fistula may develop if the colon pocket is perforated and got connected to the passage of an adjacent organ such as the bladder, which leads in turn to kidney inflammation.

Treatment

In simple cases the treatment can include antibiotics and maintaining a diet of light nutritious food and liquids.

A surgery may become necessary in severe cases, especially in cases of extreme repetitive annoying pain. The procedure involves cutting off the affected part of the colon. In some cases, a reverse colostomy is necessary to get rid of the body waste and reduce the inflammation and then the intestine are reconnected upon healing.

BLUE AMERICANS

The Fugate Family

The story of the Fugate family started with the arrival of Martin Fugate from France to Kentucky wherein he got married to Elizabeth Smith and got seven children four of them were bluish in color. The blue color was obvious on their faces and limbs. This caused the family a lot of grief for being abnormal and different from the rest of the white community. They withdrew from the society and lived away in an isolated hilly area. The family was called the Blue Fugates.

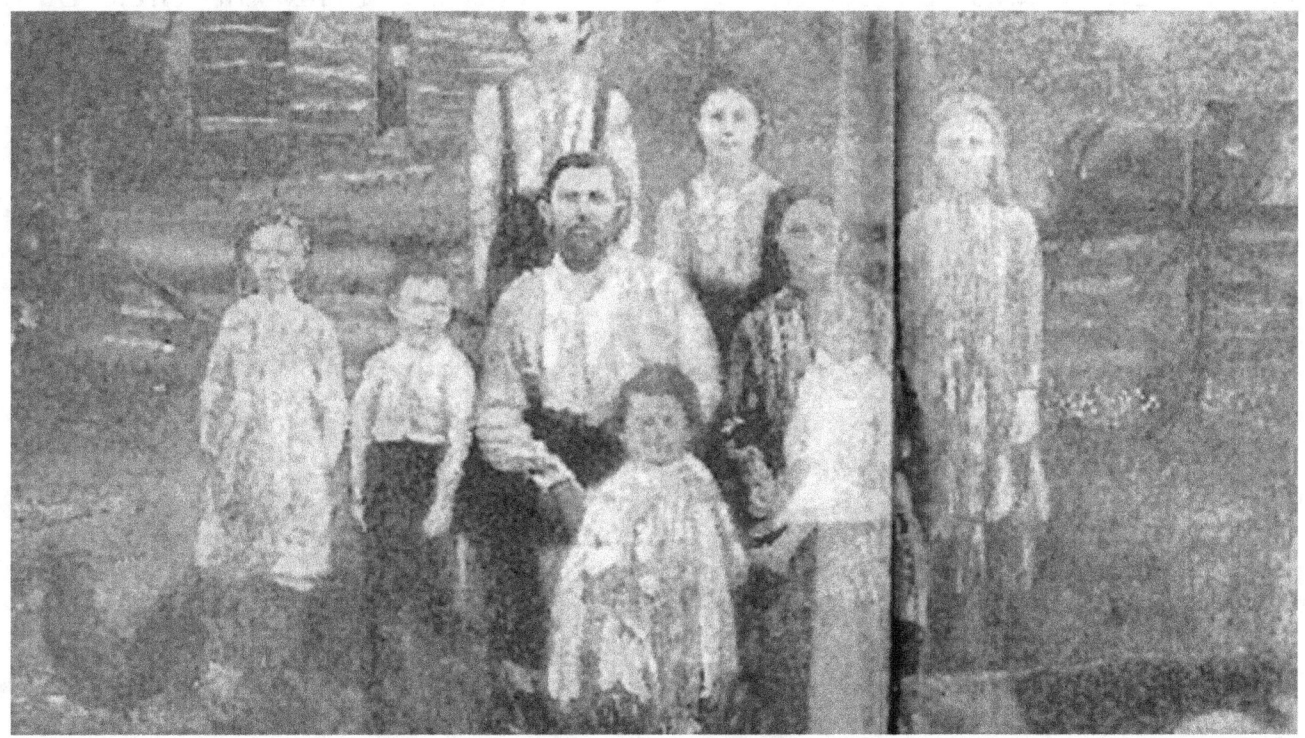

The Fugate Family

The Abnormal Hemoglobin was the Reason

The hemoglobin is a matter present in the red blood cells. The hemoglobin carries the oxygen to distribute it on the body cells. In the case of the Fugate family, there was a high percentage of hemoglobin called methemoglobin. Excess of methemoglobin in the blood is referred to as methemoglobinemia which is naturally present at a low percent that does not exceed 1%. When the percentage of methemoglobinemia rises to about 20% or more; as was the case with the Fugate family, the blood becomes incapable of carrying enough oxygen to the limbs and extremities. This causes cyanosis of the face especially the lips and the limbs especially the fingertips. Such peculiar increase in the methemoglobinemia is connected to a defective gene called Met-H, which carries recessive characteristics.

It is believed that this genetic abnormality is connected to a low level of the enzyme Cytochrome- b5 Methemoglobin Reductase, which is necessary for antioxidation of the methemoglobinemia.

In the case of the Fugates; both of the husband and the wife carried the recessive gene, which made it a common gene for the offsprings. Accordingly, the disease was transferred to the children. Eventually the circle of people carrying the disease expanded. Kentucky gained the fame by having the Blue People of Kentucky.

The Fate of the Fugate Family

It is interesting to note that members of the Fugate family survived the disease and some of them reached 80 years of age.

Gradually the offsprings of the Fugate family disappeared. The last known person from the clan was Benjamin Benly Stacy, who lived in Alaska. For all what we know, he may be still alive!

IS HIGH CHOLESTEROL HEREDITARY?

Victims of Hereditary Cholesterol

Although many years have passed, I still clearly recall the slim young man who frequented my clinic. Whenever he visited me, he had a rather sad look in his eyes. He was down on his luck as he suffered from a hereditary extremely high cholesterol, insufficiency and obstruction (clotting) in his coronary artery. The high cholesterol was spread among all his kinship and was the cause of the death of his father and brother at young age.

That was a typical case, which is medically identified as familial hypercholesterolemia (FH). Fortunately, such elevated cholesterol is rare.

How Does the Cholesterol Rise through Hereditary?

That is what takes place …

There are two types of cholesterol; a beneficial or good cholesterol called high-density lipoproteins (HDL) and a harmful type called low-density lipoproteins (LDL). It is sometimes called the "bad" cholesterol because a high LDL level leads to a buildup of cholesterol in the arteries; that may lead to a heart attack.

Each cell has a receptor made from protein. The problem arises when the LDL receptor seizes to operate and does not respond to the need of the cell for cholesterol. In this case the LDL cannot be consumed and accumulate in the arteries including the coronal artery that feeds the heart muscle. That malfunction is attributed to a deformed gene that transfers from either parent or both to their children.

When the defective gene is transferred from the father or the mother the case is called Heterozygous FH. In this case half of the LDL receptors do not work. In contrast, if the defective genes are transferred by both parents the case the case is called Monozygous FH wherein all LDL receptors cease to work, and the bad cholesterol LDL rises to a threatening level.

The Monozygous FH case is most the dangerous since the LDL exceeds 400 dl/mg and may be elevated to 1,000 dl/mg.

The Monozygous FH affects1 in 1000,000 and leads to cardiac events and to early death.

Extremely high cholesterol can precipitate on the Achilles tendon (the lower part of the leg) and other tendons. Furthermore, it precipitates around the eyes as small lumps yellowish in color.

When Do we Claim that the Elevation of Cholesterol is Related to the Genes (FH)?

Some signs that indicate that the elevation of cholesterol is attributed to inherited genes are:

- Elevation of the total cholesterol to more than 300 dl/mg.
- Elevation of the bad cholesterol (LDL) to more than 200 dl/mg.
- Cardiac arrest at young age.
- Precipitation of the cholesterol as lumps in the body, such as on the Achilles tendon or around the eyes.
- The lack of response of the cholesterol level to lowering treatments despite healthy diet that are low in fat.

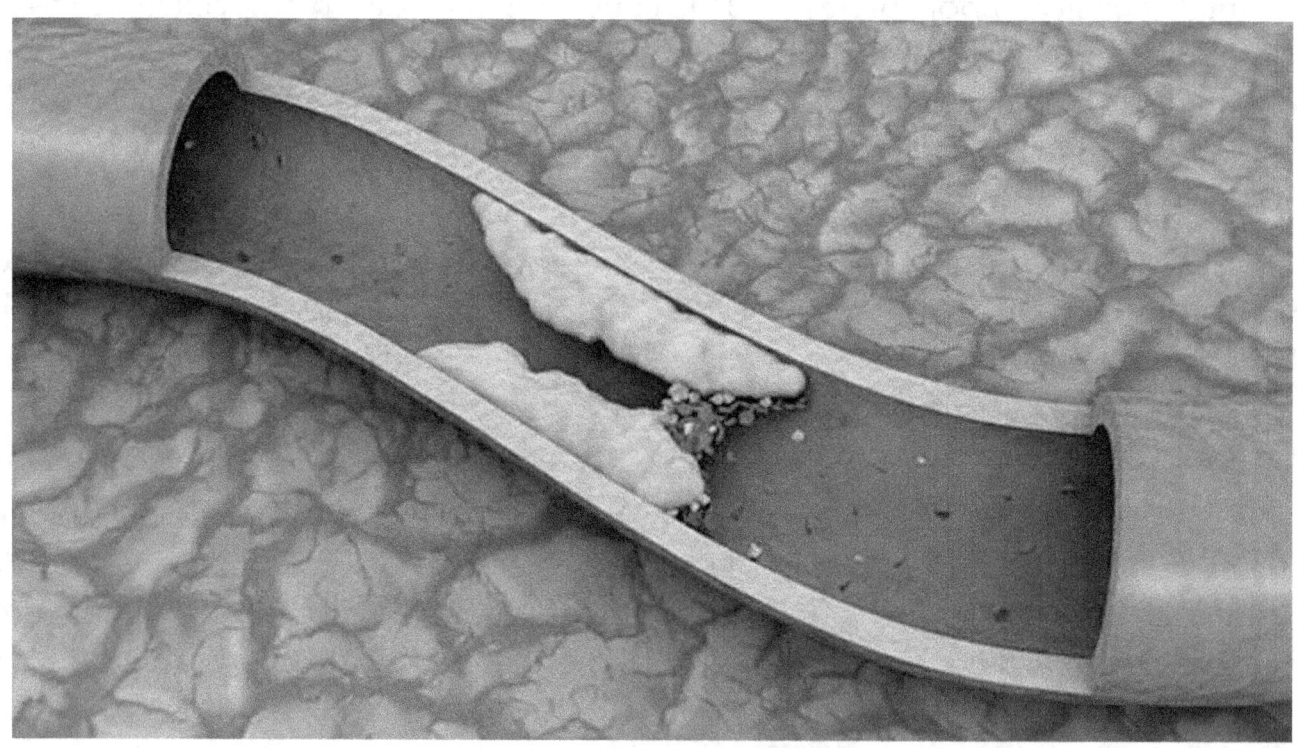

Precipitation of cholesterol in the coronary artery

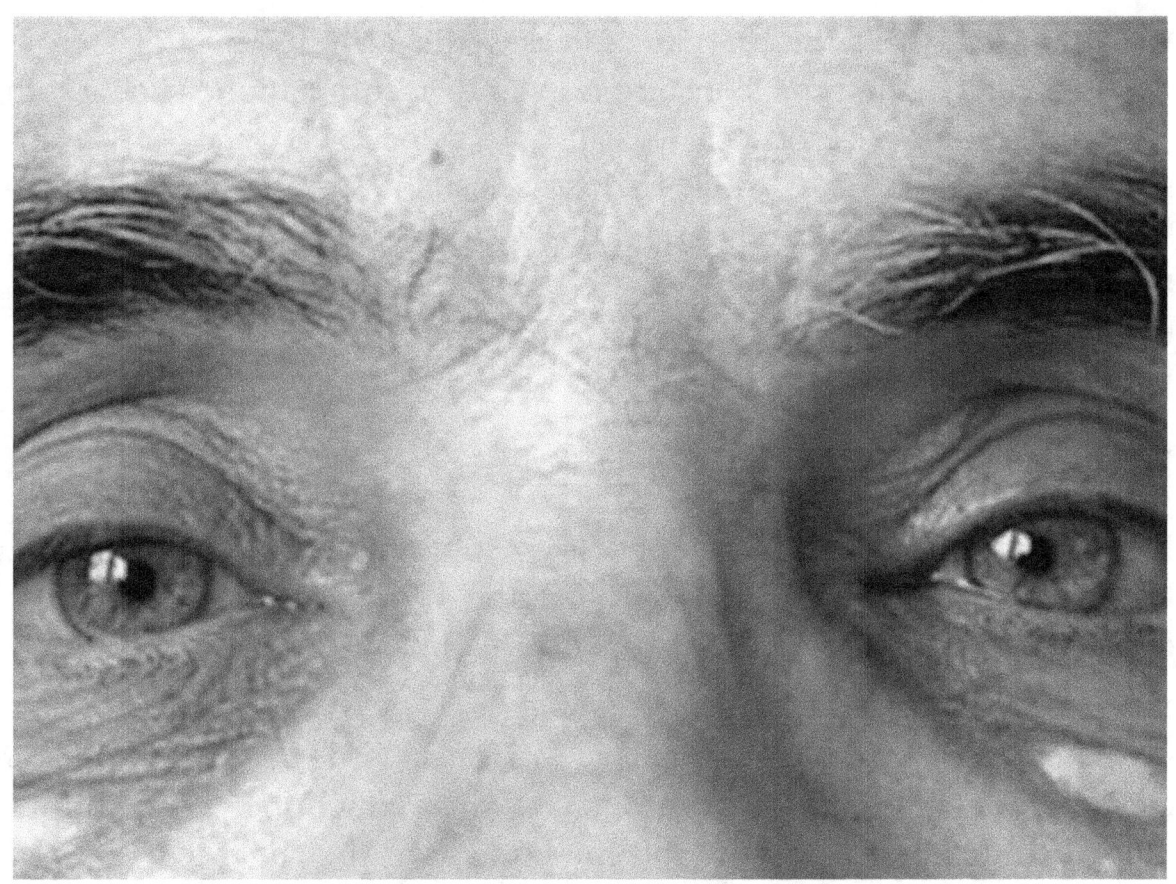

Precipitation of cholesterol around the face

When does the Chances for Elevated Cholesterol Increases in General?

The tendency to elevated cholesterol increases in the following cases:

- Obesity, especially inherited obesity wherein the fat accumulates around the chest and the stomach (round like an apple), where in the waist grows in excess of 40 inch for men and 35 for women.
- Hereditary tendency for the lever to produce large amounts of cholesterol. The normal lever produces 70% of the cholesterol, while the rest of the cholesterol is obtained through nutrition. The excessive production of cholesterol by the lever is a phenomenon spread among some families wherein the father, mother or brother have elevated cholesterol levels. This is enhanced in cases of inherited obesity.
- A diet rich with concentrated fat such as the consumption of fatty cuts of meat, whole milk and dairy products, processed sweets that is manufactured using trans fatty acids.

- Contracting diseases that increases the affinity to cholesterol elevation, since it affects its consumption and accumulation, such as the thyroid malfunctions especially Hashimoto's disease (one of the autoimmune diseases), diabetes and lever diseases such as the fatty lever.
- Administration of diuretic drugs to increase production of urine from the Thiazide type.
- Lax in physical activities
- Alcohol.

How to Treat Elevated Cholesterol?

For those who have HF, it is necessary to administer high doses of drugs that lower the cholesterol level to protect the heart and the arteries. Following a cholesterol lowering diet only is not sufficient in cases of highly elevated cholesterol levels.

In other cases, it is necessary to deal with the reasons leading to the elevation of cholesterol levels, such as the reduction in consumption of red meat, elimination of obesity, and the control of the sugar level in blood. At the same time, it is necessary to administer drugs that lower the cholesterol level with doses appropriate for the level of increase in the cholesterol level.

It is beneficial to consume high fiber nutritious foods, complex carbohydrates (high fiber) such as vegetables, fruits, whole grains and baked goods from whole grain flour. The presence of high fiber in the intestines reduces the absorption of cholesterol from the food and helps in get riding from the any excess.

It is also beneficial to consume olive oil, fatty acids that contain omega-3 which is available in fat fish such as tuna, salmon and sardines. This is in addition to consumption of moderate quantities of raw nuts that contain useful vegetable oils with unconcentrated fatty acids. Beneficial oils such as flaxseed oil is also recommended.

GOUT ... IS IT A MALE'S DISEASE?!

Statistics

If you are a male, you would have a high affinity to have gout compared to females. If you also have a family history perceptive to gout, your chances of getting gout are rather high.

Through observation of patients that patron clinics, including my clinic, it is hard to find a female complaining of gout.

In a clinical statistical study, it was found that the chances of males suffering from gout are 10 times more than females.

A hereditary factor was found for having gout; nevertheless, there was no specific gene identified as the reason.

In addition to the fact that gout is more prevalent among men than women, gout is more prevalent among some families at a high rate. This explains the fact that some people are likely to have gout more than others although both consume a great deal of meat, which is a factor for promoting gout.

But, Why ... ?

The most pronounced difference between males and females is mainly in the difference in hormones which specifies the traits of masculinity and femininity.

It is most likely that the femininity hormones called estrogen provides the necessary protection against gout. Accordingly, it can be noticed that most gout cases among women occur after reaching the menopause which is accompanied by the end of production of estrogen by the ovaries. The presence of estrogen at a natural level prevent the increase in the level of uric acid, which is responsible for gout. Such benefit is not available to males. Nevertheless, the ratio of men contracting gout remains higher than women, even if women has reached their menopause.

Why Was Gout Called the Royal Disease?

Contracting gout is related to the elevation of the uric acid level due to the decomposition of food rich in purine. The most prominent among purine-rich foods is meat which is the main food staple of the rich and the royalties. This is how the disease became known as the royal disease.

In realty gout is the disease of the poor as well, since purine is plentiful in cheap and more affordable food staple, such as legumes, dry beans and lentils.

One of the most famous celebrities who had gout was Suleiman the Lawgiver (aka Suleiman the Magnificent in the West) the Sultan of the Ottoman Empire (1520-1566). Although he suffered from the painful disease, he was able to expand the Empire.

Why does Gout Affect the Joints and the Mobility?

Gout is also called Gouty Arthritis since it causes inflammation in the joints.

When the body fails to rid of the excess uric acid through urination, the uric acid crystals which are shaped like thin needles get deposited in the joints and the surrounding tissues causing swelling inflammation, pain, and redness.

Such complications can take place in different joints such as the knee and the ankle. However, it tends to act more strenuously on the big toes which affect the individual's gait and mobility.

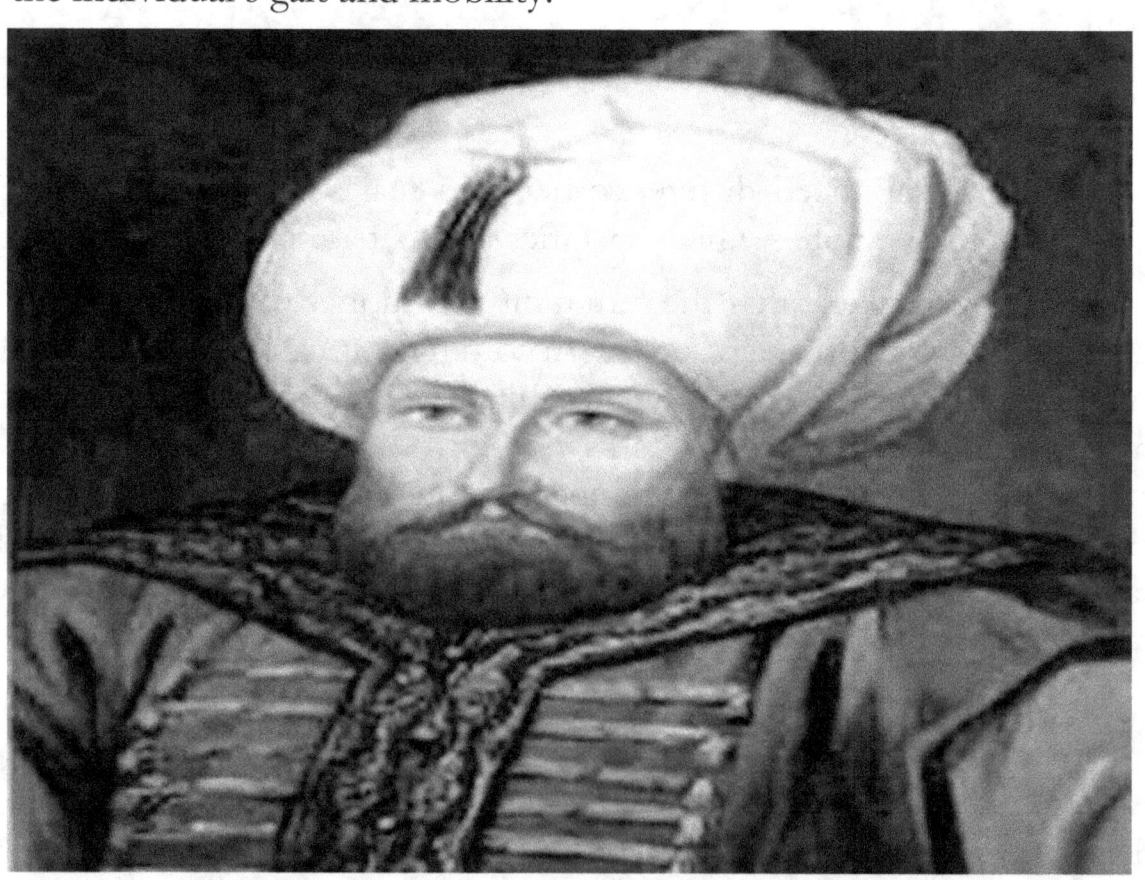

Suleiman the Lawgiver (Suleiman the Magnificent in the West) Sultan of the Ottoman Empire

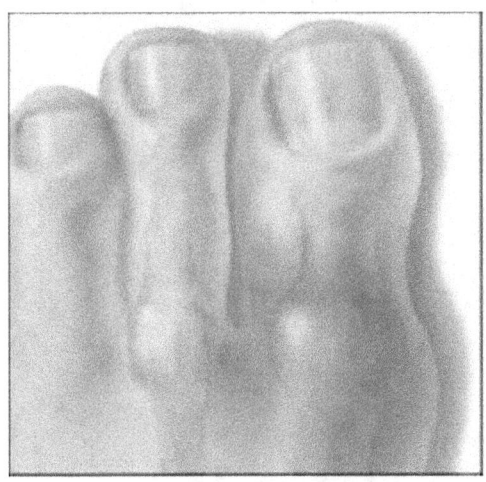

Big toe suffering from intense gout

Acute and Chronic Gout

The gout could attack the body in a sudden episode that wakes the person from deep sleep on severe pain due to swelling and redness of the toes. With proper treatment the case gradually improves, and the pain diminishes. Anti-inflammatory medications such as colchicine (Common brands: Mitigare, Colcrys) can treat and prevent gout attacks. However, that does not reduce the uric acid in the blood stream. Accordingly, the formation of the uric acid crystals continues and so is there deposits in the joints. The disease can turn into chronic disease unless care is continued after each episode by further medication to lower the level of the uric acid by reducing its production in the body. This is in addition to other treatments to get rid of the excess uric acid through urination.

In the chronic situations the pain become less severe, however, the uric acid precipitation as crystals may lead to formation of tophi (stones) deposits. Tophi are pathognomonic for the disease gout. Longstanding high levels of uric acid in the blood is a condition known as hyperuricemia.

The Healing Cherry Dish

A man was suffering from gout felt great intolerable pain. To get his mind off the excruciating pain he entertained himself by munching on cherries from a large dish filled with cherry. Amazingly, he started to feel better. Since then the cherry gained the fame as a means of alleviating the pain from the gout, if consumed in large quantities.

It is interesting also, that some studies connected between the daily coffee drinking and the reduction of uric acid in the blood. Nevertheless, there is no explanation of such connection until now.

WHY DO BLADDER INFLAMMATION AND BURNING URINATION PROBLEMS PREVAIL AMONG WOMEN MORE THAN MEN?!

Disturbing Symptoms

If you suffer from the frequent need to urinate, but only small amounts of urine are passed each time and yet you have pressing urges to urinate while you feel unable to hold it then you have cystitis, that is inflammation of the bladder wall. Cystitis also entails burning sensation during urination, especially towards the end (due to shrinking of the bladder).

Cystitis affects people of both sexes and all ages. It is more common among females than males due to anatomical differences; that is because women have shorter urethras. Accordingly, the female is most susceptible to bladder infection if she does not take more stringent precautions.

Here is the Explanation …

The urethral opening and the vagina opening are remarkably close. This makes it easily for the vagina to get infected and any microbes around it can easily reach the urethral opening. In addition, the female's urethra is rather short compared to the male which make it easy for germs to reach the bladder.

Beware of the Common Mistake!

Among the common mistakes that females subconsciously do during washing or drying the vagina is to move the hand from the back to the top that is from the vaginal opening or from the anus towards the urethral opening. This can easily transfer any present bacteria or waste to the urethral opening. Subsequently, these pathogens will find their way to the bladder causing inflammation of the bladder.

In the same time negligence in cleaning the vagina generally leads to contamination of the urethral opening.

In order to avoid inflammation of the bladder; and especially repeated or frequent inflammation it is necessary to clean the vagina with keen care and use hand strokes from the vagina back and not up. It is also recommended to wear cotton underwear because underwear made from synthetic fibers does not allow airing of that area which promotes multiplication of the bacteria. It is also preferred to avoid scented preparations, including sprays in the vicinity of the vagina. The use of bubble path and other chemical formulations can irritate the bladder opening and promote inflammation.

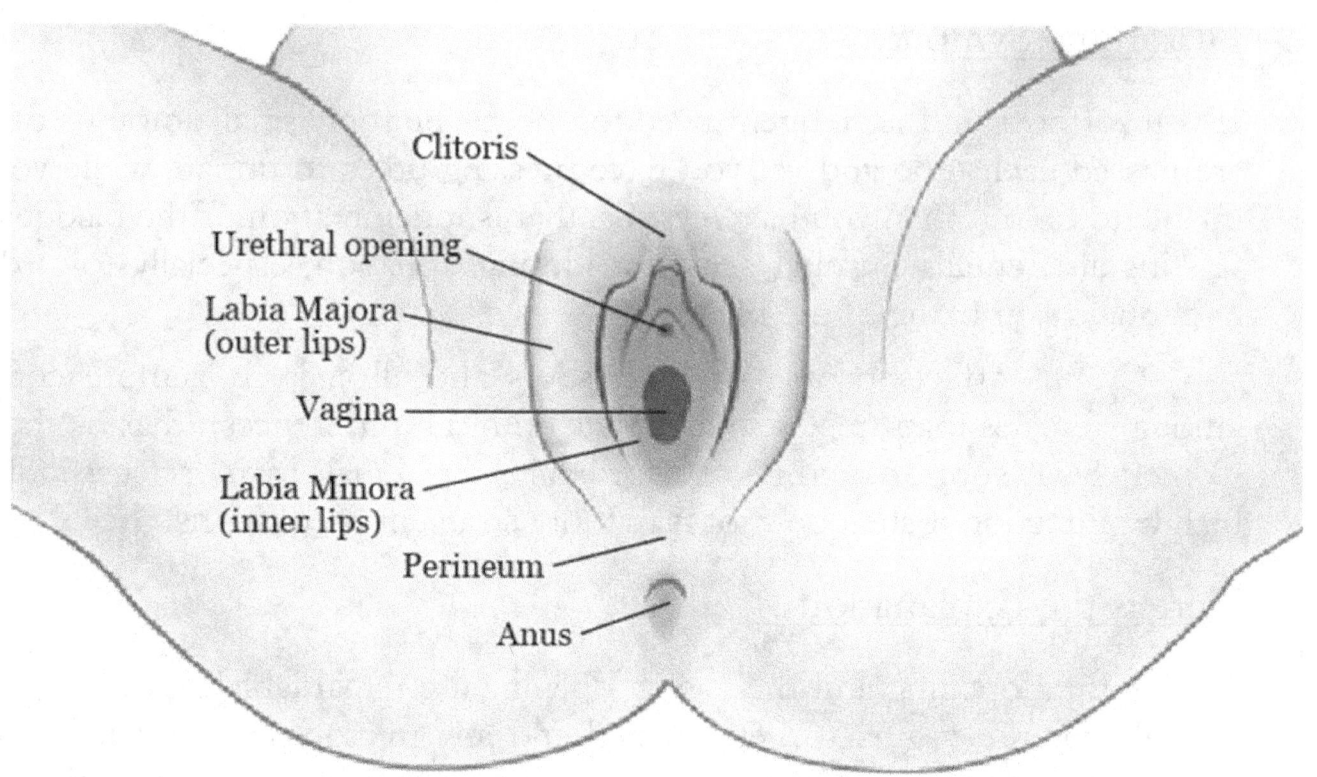

The Type of Bacteria

In many situations the infection by Escherichia coli (E. coli) can take place. It is interesting to know that this bacterium lives peacefully in the intestine. However, when it moves to the bladder it becomes pathogenic. This is exactly what happens when these bacteria are transferred from the anus to the vagina during the wrong way of cleaning the vagina after defecation.

Honeymoon Inflammation!

The inflammation of the bladder in females may be connected to sexual intercourse, especially during the initial period of marriage in what is known as honeymoon cystitis. The cause of that is repeated intercourse without proper washing following each round. This can lead to microbial contamination of vaginal secretion or sperm fluid.

Treatment

The inflammation of the bladder can be treated by the appropriate antibiotics for the necessary period according to the advice of the physician. It is also necessary to consume plenty of water and fluids.

WHEN DOES THE CHANCES INCREASE FOR CONTRACTING THE MEDITERRANEAN ANEMIA?

Thalassemia

The Mediterranean anemia is called thalassemia which indicates the lack of blood.

This type of anemia is connected to the Mediterranean Sea because it is widely spread among the countries around the Mediterranean Sea, including Egypt, Cyprus, Greece and Italy. However, this anemia is present in many other countries far away from the Mediterranean Sea, such as East Asia.

In addition to the actual prevalence of this disease among the Nations located around the Mediterranean Sea, the percentage of those who carry the gene connected to thalassemia without displaying the symptoms is about 10%.

What Causes this Anemia?

The cause of thalassemia is related to the formation of abnormal hemoglobin, which is present in the red blood cells and is responsible for carrying the oxygen to the body cells.

The hemoglobin is the combination of two words: the word heme which is an iron-containing compound of the porphyrin class which forms the nonprotein part of hemoglobin and some other biological molecules. The second word is globin which is a protein comprise of two types of protein, alpha and beta. The defect in the hemoglobin resides in the abnormality of the protein which in the case of the disease is compromised of only one of those two proteins. This is caused by a defective gene that is inherited by the children from their parents.

What are the Consequences?

In the case of thalassemia, the hemoglobin does not transfer adequate quantity of oxygen to the body cells. At the same time, the life of the red blood cells is short. However, the worst repercussion from that is the destruction of the red blood cells, since they carry a type of hemoglobin which is strange to the body. Accordingly, the immune system starts to attack that alien substance and destroy it. Such destruction or dissolution leads to the separation of the iron from the heme and its accumulation in the blood stream. The iron gets deposited in the organs including the heart, the liver and the brains. Furthermore, the hemoglobin after leaving the blood gets converted to bilirubin. Bilirubin is a yellow compound that occurs in the normal catabolic pathway that breaks down heme from hemoglobin, myoglobin, peroxidases, and cytochromes. This catabolism is a necessary process in the body's clearance of waste products that arise from the destruction of aged or abnormal red blood cells.

The bilirubin dyes the skin and the sclera (aka the white of the eye) yellowish color. The urine becomes dark yellow or brown. The affected person face will be pale yellow as and outcome of jaundice (icterus); which is a medical condition with yellowing of the skin or whites of the eyes, arising from excess of the pigment bilirubin and typically caused by obstruction of the bile duct, by liver disease, or by excessive breakdown of red blood cells.

How does The Mediterranean Anemia Get Inherited?

This disease carries the recessive characteristic however if it is combined with an identical gene it will assume a dominant characteristic promoting a chance of infecting or not infecting the offspring, as follows:

If a disease carrying man got married to a disease carrying woman; that is if both have a defective gene without showing the symptoms of the disease, the outcome will be:

- Conception of a child with the disease: 25%.
- Conception of a child carrying the disease: 50%.
- Conception of a healthy child: 25%.

When does the Chance of a Child Born with the Disease Increase?

Marriage between relatives increases the chance of infecting a child or more with disease due to an increase of the probability of the presence of the defective gene in both parties.

Types of Thalassemia

There are two types of Thalassemia (it may be divided in 3 types as well): thalassemia minor and thalassemia major and the difference between both types is great.

Thalassemia Minor

In the thalassemia minor, the child carries the defective gene from either parent, when one of them is carrying the defective gene while the other is healthy.

In this case the symptoms are not clear, and the disease carrier lives his/her life naturally and worry free or some minor symptoms may show such as the red blood spheres are small or the hemoglobin level does nor exceed 10 mg despite of a healthy diet.

Thalassemia Major

The thalassemia major is severe anemia distinct by clear symptoms and severe repercussions, as follows:

- Slow growth.
- Paleness and yellowish complexions.
- Dyspnea (shortness of breath) and getting tired fast for the least effort.
- Blueish lips (due to oxygen insufficiency).
- Enlargement of the spleen (since it is the organ that filters the blood and collects broken and spoiled red blood cells) and in extreme cases the spleen may be removed.
- Enlargement of the lever in addition to the enlargement of the spleen leading to general enlargement of the stomach.
- Deformation of the bones such as expansion of the bones and may lead to macrocephaly (overly large head).
- Problems with the heart, the brains or other organs due to the accumulation of iron in the blood and deposition in different organs; the increase in iron could be a killer.

When will the Symptoms of the Thalassemia Major Appear?

The Symptoms of this type of dangerous thalassemia (thalassemia major) appear after about 6 months from birth. This is because the child relies on the hemoglobin obtained from his/her mother's body before that time. Then the child starts to produce new abnormal hemoglobin.

In the following period the mother notices paleness of the child's complexions and irregular growth. The mother needs to consult with a physician at that time.

How Can the Mediterranean Anemia be Diagnosed?

In addition to the appearance of the symptoms of the disease, the case can be diagnosed through a complete blood count (CBC) wherein the hemoglobin level will be low (around 7 mg).

To determine the defect in the hemoglobin an electrophoresis has to be conducted on the hemoglobin. Electrophoresis is the motion of dispersed particles relative to a fluid under the influence of a spatially uniform electric field.

What is the Treatment of the Mediterranean Anemia?

The thalassemia major requires frequent blood transfusion. Nevertheless, repeated blood transfusion will cause a rise in the iron level in the blood over the already hard level. This will constitute great harm. Accordingly, blood transfusion must be combined with administration of drugs to reduce the iron level in the blood.

The straightforward treatment is the bone marrow transplant which yields good results.

Prevention

Giving birth to a child with thalassemia major causes an extraordinary psychological burden on the parents let alone the enormous cost in childcare.

It is advisable to conduct a genetic test on the couple who intend to marry. This is absolutely necessary for those who intend to marry close relatives.

It is also possible to conduct a genetic test on the fetus during pregnancy. If the test was positive the pregnancy must be terminated in the first trimester.

WHO ARE THOSE MOST SUSCEPTIBLE TO THE MEDITERRANIAN FEVER?

How do the Symptoms of the Disease Appear?

Most of the cases of Familial Mediterranean Fever (FMF) that I came across through my practice as a physician were suffering from excoriating ache in the stomach that makes the patient writhing from the intolerable pain in addition to a slight elevation in the temperature. Nevertheless, there are other cases that suffered much more. The patient does not have to show all the symptoms. In addition to stomachache and rise in temperature the patient may also complain from:

- Chest pain.
- Join pain and swelling (the knee, specially).
- Muscles pain (specially legs' muscles) without exerting any effort.
- Possible appearance of rash especially on the legs.
- Possible swelling in the scrotum or inflammation in the testicles.

Potential Complications

The pain in the joint can become chronic. The reproductive organs, especially in women, may suffer from the disease repercussions including inability to conceive or sterility. The disease may lead to abnormal increase in the Amyloid-A body protein which would deposit in the body organs leading to amyloidosis which is dangerous. If the protein deposits in the kidney; for example, it may eventually lead to renal failure accompanied with appearance of protein in the urine.

Painful Episodes

The FMF disease ordinarily starts at childhood. The most distinct features of the disease are that it takes place in episodes that differ in intensity and frequency. In many cases the episodes are limited to stomachache which is most often severe.

The pain is attributed to Peritonitis, the inflammation of the serous membrane lining the abdominal wall and covering the abdominal organs (peritoneum). Ordinarily the pain commences at a part of the stomach and spreads to the rest of the stomach. It lasts for a period that ranges from one to three days. This is followed by a healthy period that may last for a month or two. Then, the episode is repeated one or two times yearly. This is why those who suffers from the familial Mediterranean fever are aware very well of the symptoms of the episodes and how to handle them by relieving drugs.

Treatment

There is no assured treatment for FMF. Accordingly, the means of prevention of the episodes have a great weight. Colchicine is known to reduce the frequency of the episodes and ease the pain.

Since Colchicine is a poisonous formulation it is necessary to use a limited dose under the supervision of the physician which must periodically review the treatment and health status. This is rather important since the patient has to use the drug through lifetime and not only when needed or during the episodes.

The physician usually prescribes antiinflammation non-cortisone drugs to fight the inflammation and reduce the pain.

Laboratory Tests

The following laboratory tests have to be performed periodically:
- Amyloid A level: high
- CBC: high count of white blood cells because of the inflammation case.

When does the Chances of Contracting the Disease Increase?

- The familial Mediterranean fever is known to spread among certain families. The infection of members of a family by the disease increases the chance of infection of other family members.
- The defective gene is passed on through generations in a recessive manner; that is the individual who has the gene does not necessarily show the symptom of the disease. The person is considered only as a carrier. However, when the gene is transferred from the father and the mother to the child the defective gene became a common gene among the offsprings.
- Marriage from close relatives or next of kin increases the possibility of the disease to the offspring.

- The likelihood of having familial Mediterranean fever among the population in the region is high. However, the disease may be contracted by the Turkish and Armenian population.

Prevention

It is possible to conduct diagnosis to identify the defective gene related to the familial Mediterranean fever; that is MEFV, especially among members of families that have been affected by FMF. The test must be done before marriage although avoiding the marriage of close relatives or bringing up children if the marriage took place is an advisable way to prevent the spread of the disease.

DIFFICULTIES OF THE THYROID, THE WOMEN'S FRIEND!

The Reasons

The gender factor clearly appears in encountering thyroid difficulties and the inheritance factor plays an important role as well.

The percentage of having thyroid problems among women is about ten times the occurrence among women. The question is why?

The most important reason is the hormonic changes in the female body which is related to the monthly period. This is in addition to the propensity to inherit the thyroid difficulties due to the fact that such problems are more prevalent among specific families than others. Also, it is believed that the frequent change in the mode and the inclination to agitation play a role in that matter.

Where is the Thyroid?

The Thyroid is a butterfly-shaped endocrine gland consisting of two connected lobes, connected by a bridge (isthmus) in the middle. It sits low on the front of the neck below Adam's apple and along the front of the windpipe. Brownish-red in color, the thyroid is rich with blood vessels.

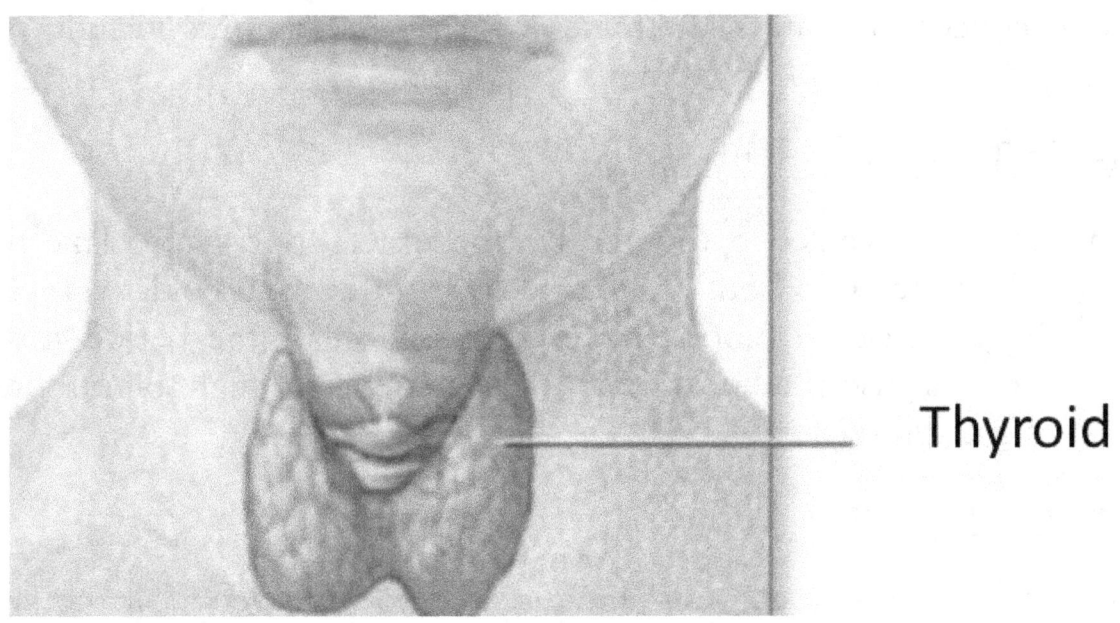

The thyroid secretes several hormones, collectively called thyroid hormones. The main thyroid hormone is thyroxine (T_4), triiodothyronine (T_3) and a peptide hormone, calcitonin. Secretion of the two thyroid hormones (T_3, T_4) is regulated by the thyroid-stimulating hormone (TSH), which is secreted from the anterior pituitary gland. TSH is regulated by thyrotropin-releasing hormone (TRH), which is produced by the hypothalamus. Nerves important for voice quality also pass through the thyroid.

Thyroid hormones act throughout the body, influencing metabolism and protein synthesis, growth and development, and body temperature. Calcitonin plays a role in calcium homeostasis.

Weakness of Thyroid Activity

Reasons for Weight Increase May be Connected to Thyroid!

Hypothyroidism (a condition in which the thyroid gland doesn't produce enough thyroid hormone) weakens the metabolism and food digestion which lead to storage of the fat in the body and increase in weight. Hypothyroidism's deficiency of thyroid hormones results in sapping energy at all levels. It can disrupt such things as heart rate, body temperature, and all aspects of metabolism.

Major symptoms of hypothyroidism include fatigue, cold sensitivity, constipation, dry skin, and unexplained weight gain. This is in addition to inability to concentrate and forgetfulness. Physical symptoms include swelling and sagging of eye lids and heavy menstrual blood.

Increase in Thyroid Activity

The symptoms of overactive thyroid are the exact opposite of lazy thyroid. Those include decrease in body weight, feeling hot even in cold weather, rapid heartbeat, light menstrual blood and even cessation of the period for a few months. There is also the possibility of experiencing high blood pressure, bulging eyes and diarrhea.

Hashimoto's Disease

Hashimoto's disease is an autoimmune disease and is named after the Japanese physician Hakaru Hashimoto best known for publishing the first description of the disease that would later be named Hashimoto's thyroiditis (aka chronic lymphocytic thyroiditis).

As most autoimmune diseases, the Hashimoto's disease is likely to target females. It gradually destroys the thyroid gland. Early on there may be no symptoms. Over time the thyroid may enlarge, forming a painless goiter leading to throat tightness or trouble breathing. Some people eventually develop hypothyroidism with accompanying weight gain, feeling tired, constipation, depression and general pains. The level of cholesterol may rise. After many years the thyroid typically shrinks in size. Potential complications include thyroid lymphoma.

Hashimoto's thyroiditis is thought to be due to a combination of genetic and environmental factors. The likelihood of contracting the increases is the presence of another autoimmune diseases, such as:

- Type 1 diabetes.
- Systemic Lupus Erythematosus (SLE).
- Joint rheumatoid.
- Vitiligo

Risk factors include a family history of the condition. This is evidenced by the presence of the disease among family members. However, no specific gene is identified which is connected to Hashimoto's thyroiditis.

How we can Treat Thyroid Problems?

In addition to the symptoms of hyperthyroidism and hypothyroidism, diagnosis can confirm the situation through blood tests for TSG, T4, and anti-thyroid autoantibodies.

In the case of hypothyroidism, the treatment can be through administering synthesized thyroxin hormones with a limited dose to be subscribed by a physician.

In the case of hyperthyroidism, the treatment involves administering drugs that slows the thyroid activity. However, some patients may require the removal of a part of the thyroid. Also, radioactive iodine may be used to destroy the active tissues of the thyroid.

The anticipated drawbacks of surgery are lowering the thyroid activity by removal of a large tissue of the thyroid which has to be compensated by makeup hormones the rest of the life. The surgery may also affect the focal cords since the thyroid is very close to the voice box, or larynx.

The Most Famous People Affected by Thyroid Problems

One of the most famous figures who suffered from hyperthyroidism is the popular classical Egyptian singer Um Kalthoom. She was forced to wear dark glasses even at night to hide the bulge in her eyes. She refused surgery in fear of affecting her vocal cord.

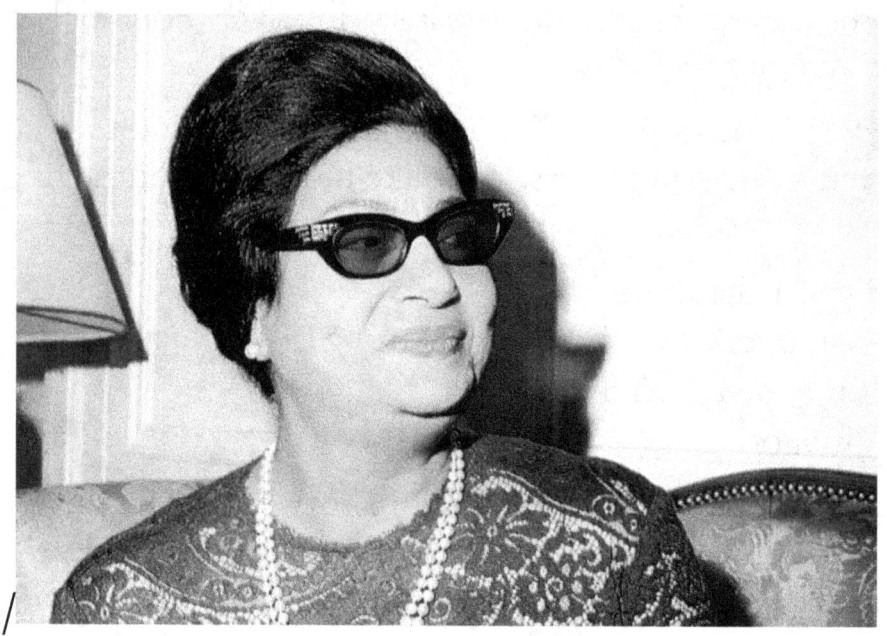

Um Kalthoom

FACTORS THAT ENHANCE THE LIKELIHOOD OF GALLBLADER TROUBLES

Women are More Susceptible to Gallblader Trouble

Through my medical studies, experience and gained expertise I got to learn that the chances of development of gallbladder problems whether inflammation or formation of stones are increased in the presence of 4F: Female, Fertile, Fat, Filthy.

Where is the Gallbladder and What its Function?

The gallbladder is a 7 to10 cm (about four-inch), small elongated pear-shaped pouch. The organ sits just under the liver (on the right side of the top of the belly).

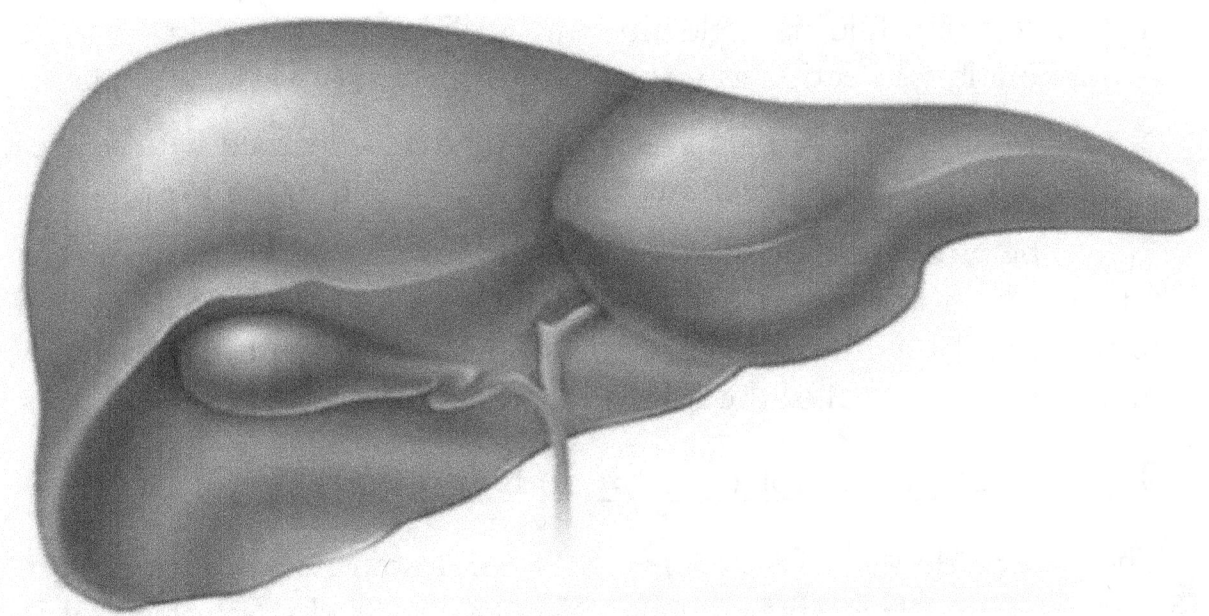

Gallbladder

The main function of the gallbladder is to store the bile, produced by the liver. During consumption of the food, the gallbladder squeezes the bile that composes and digests the fat.

The bile is squeezed through to the cystic duct and then to the common bile duct which leads to the small intestine or more accurately to the duodenum.

Gallbladder Inflammation

It is most likely that you have an inflammation of the gallbladder you are suffering from:

- Stomachache or frequent pain on the top of the right side of the belly under the ribs immediately after eating, especially if you have consumed a fatty meal or fried food.
- The pain may shoot to the right shoulder towards the top of back between the blades of the shoulders.
- Bloating, indigestion and nausea.
- Discomfort after eating and a relative ease when fasting.

Such difficulties are indicative of chronic cholecystitis which results from inflammation of the lining of the gallbladder and could be indicative of the presence of stones.

Alternatively, one may suffer from acute cholecystitis which is connected to movement of gallbladder stone and possible plugging of the cystic duct. In this case, the bile is held in the gallbladder wherein it is exposed to contamination, infection as well as the formation of waste and pus.

At that stage, the pain is severe and is accompanied with nausea, vomiting, and high temperature which may necessitate going to the hospital.

The inflammation can be treated by special medications to resist the inflammation and aid in the flow of the bile and prevent its accumulation for prevention from the formation of stones. Acute pain associated with stones may require removal of the gallbladder.

When does the Gallbladder Stone Deposits Increase?

The gallbladders are formed from the cholesterol and other matter. However, there is no evidence that the elevation of the level of cholesterol in the blood promotes the formation of the gallbladder stoned. However, the following increase the chances for stone formation in the gallbladder:

- Obesity,
- Sudden weight loss in diets designed for weight loss,
- Diabetes,
- Excess consumption of fat and fried food,

- Administration of drugs containing estrogen such as birth control pills.

What is the Danger of Gallbladder Stones?

It is surprising that the gallbladder stones may stay still in place and causes no pain and if discovered will be by mere chance.

Whenever the stones move and plug the cystic duct causing the accumulation of stagnant bile. That my lead to infection, acute pain and formation of pus.

If the stone moves to the common bile duct, the bile will return back to the liver causing obstructive jaundice which will dye the skin and the eye whites with yellowish color.

Some drugs can be used to dissolve tiny stones; nevertheless, the removal of the gallbladder assures the eradication of stones and frequent problems.

WHY FEMALES ARE MORE SUSCIPTIBLE TO OSTEOPOROSIS?

What is Osteoporosis?

I recall very well an old lady who came for a check up in my clinic. She was complaining of a chest pain centered in one location and it gets sharper with eat each inhale. When I asked her to take a deep breath, I noticed how the pain became immense. This episode immediately followed catching cold and coughing. Reviewing her chest x-ray I discovered a crack in one of her ribs. I referred her to a bone specialist.

This is an example of an osteoporosis case, which was caused by a simple common cold. The cough could have cause serious fracture.

Osteoporosis is a word means "porous bone". Viewed under a microscope, healthy bone looks like a honeycomb. That is the mineral content of the bone tissues; especially the calcium reaches a low level and the bone density drops to an extent that the bones become fragile and weak and can be easily fractured.

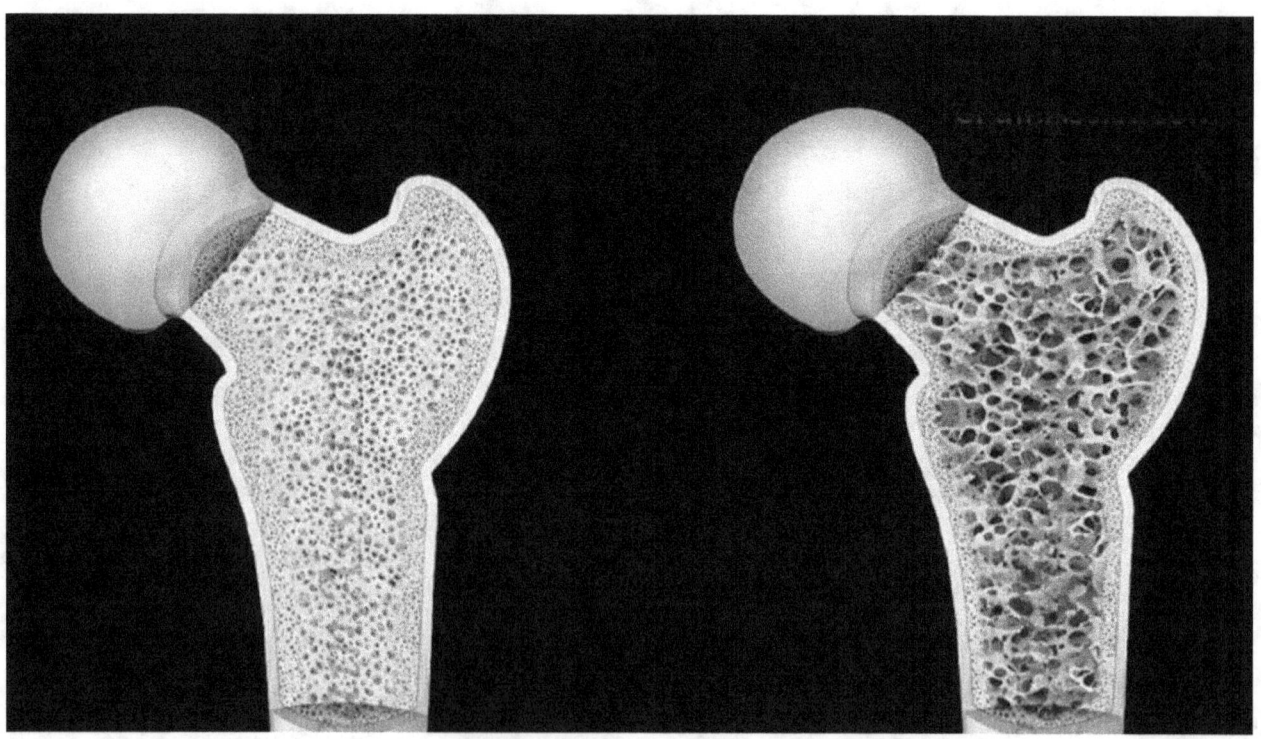

Regular bone (left) and porous bone (right)

When does the Chance of Osteoporosis Increase?

The bones pass by a natural destruction and reconstruction process wherein the older bone tissues decompose and get replaced by newer stronger tissues. This process is very active at young age. As one gets older the destruction dominates the renewal and the bones get weaker. Accordingly aging itself increase the chance for osteoporosis. The signs for that is hunch back among the elderly and the ease of breaking the bones from simple accidents.

Females are more prone to have osteoporosis at a higher percentage than males and at a younger age. This is attributed to the cessation of the menstruation period and production of the primary female sex hormone, estrogen from the ovaries upon reaching the menopause which starts in the late forties.

In that case the bone mass is reduced due to higher rate of destruction process than the rate of construction since the provision of the estrogen hormones at a normal rate is necessary for the deposition of calcium in the bones and hence the maintenance of their strength.

This problem can take place in males at an advanced age because of reduction of the testosterone hormone. However, this takes place at a percentage lower than the women and at an age over 70 years.

There is also another important factor that reduces the bones mass and reduces their strength for females as well as males. This is the sedentary lifestyle which leads to a destruction rate higher than the reconstruction rate.

Other Factors that Promote Bones Weakness and Fragility

It was determined that the negligence of supplying the body with sufficient amount of calcium and vitamin D which is necessary to absorb the calcium during the twenties and thirties of age or most precisely in the age range from 25 to 35 years reduces the individual's reserve from the bone tissues. This promotes bones weakness, porosity or fragility (osteoporosis).

The heredity factor plays a role developing osteoporosis if either parent, sister or brother has osteoporosis or if any of them suffered from fractured bone for a minor accident or injury.

The build of the body skeleton may also play a role in promoting osteoporosis. Chances of having osteoporosis in huge bodies compared to slim people with little body due to limit on the bone mass.

Hyperactive thyroid, a disease widely spread among females more than male impacts the osteoporosis. Excess secretion of the thyroxine hormone affects the loss of bone mass. The same problem arises in case of hypoactive thyroid which requires administration of thyroxine hormone. The higher the dose the more prone the person to osteoporosis.

Administration of cortisone drugs tend to harm the bone tissues if taken in high doses of cortisone over long periods of time. Examples are antidepressants that lead to increase the levels of serotonin in the brains, Selective Serotonin Reuptake Inhibitor (SSRI); such as Prozac.

Among the lifestyle effects on enhancing the presence of osteoporosis are excessive smoking. The caffeine in coffee, tea, cocoa, dark soda (cola) reduces the absorption of calcium.

- Osteoporosis Symptoms
- Hunch back,
- Shrinking of height,
- Repeated bone fracture in minor incidents,
- Back pain that may be cause by crack, fracture, or collapse of some bony vertebrae.

Measurement of Bone Density

Measurement of bone density is a necessary and important to identify the strength of the bones. It is advised that such measurement be made as the age progresses or when there is a high propensity for osteoporosis. The measurement is achieved by a test called DEXA, wherein the absorption of x-rays by the bones is measured. The test can be done in a short time.

The test is performed on the bone locations that are more prone to porosity which is wrist and hip bones.

The test reveals two aspects: osteopenia and osteoporosis. The reduction in bone mass density, which is called osteopenia, a stage precedes osteoporosis. Osteopenia requires taking all precautions and protection to avoid osteoporosis.

Treatment

Lately there are drugs that delay the loss of bone mass. In addition, it is necessary to administer calcium and vitamin D preparations as well as assuring consumption of food rich in calcium and vitamin D.

Calcium is plentiful in milk and dairy products. Yogurt has higher content of calcium than milk per serving. Food rich in calcium include leafy vegetables such as celery and parsley. Also, fish bones are rich in calcium. Small bony fish can be eaten with the bones.

Furthermore, vitamin D is available in fortified milk, egg yolk, fish oil. The body can synthesize vitamin D through exposure to sun rays.

Does Estrogen Benefit in Prevention of Osteoporosis?

That is true … It us possible to compensate for deficiency in the estrogen hormone by taking is in a synthesized form. Nevertheless, this may involve harmful strong side effects. Therefore, such hormone treatment is not common.

It is also possible to acquire estrogenic matter, that has the same effect as estrogen, and consume the food rich in such matter, such as soybeans and its products.

WHEN DOES THE CHANCE FOR HAVING RHEUMATOID DISEASE INCREASE?

Danger Factors

The percentage of contracting the rheumatoid disease among females is much higher than males. I have noticed that fact through my examination of my patients in my clinic. To my regret that most of those complaining from the rheumatoid disease are relatively young. Some were still in their twenties. Because most of the rheumatoid disease patients were females made me remember very well the faces and names of men having rheumatoid disease since they were much fewer.

Also, I got to learn from my conversations with the patients that they suffer from extreme psychological stress. This plays a major role in having rheumatoid disease. The contrary was also true. That is the psychological stress-free state plays a role in helping the patient confront the disease and ease its symptoms and repercussions. Such state is affected by the people surrounding the patient as well as the living environment.

There could be an inherited predisposition to the rheumatoid disease, since acquiring the disease could be repetitive in the same family. However, there is no specific recessive gene that can be identified with this disease.

The statistics show that obesity plays a role in promoting the rheumatoid disease. Nevertheless, I have not witnessed that in my clinical experience!

What Happens in Rheumatoid Disease?

In rheumatoid disease, the body turns on itself. In other words, the disease attacks the immune system. More precisely it attacks the synovial membranes that pads some of the joints. This is why it is classified as one of the autoimmune diseases. In a sense the rheumatoid disease is like lupus (SLE) which is also contracted by more females than males.

The reason behind the mistakes of the immune system are not clear. It could take place due to prior virus infection, especially Epstein Barr virus.

The rheumatoid disease severely affects the joints and interferes with the patient's mobility. The disease affects other patient's organs such as the heart, the lungs, the blood vessels and the skin.

The rheumatoid disease comes in attacks or episodes that can be severe and devastating followed by a period of reemission. Humidity and extreme cold triggers the episodes. This is other than the effect of the psychological conditions.

Symptoms

- Tender, warm, swollen joints: The rheumatoid disease starts at the fingers and hands. The same joint is affected by the disease on both sides of the body. This is one of the distinctive characteristics of the rheumatoid disease when compared to other ailments of the joints.
- Stiffness of the joints: The patients have hard time moving the affected joint. They can no longer stretch their fingers or get out of bed before an hour or more. This recurs every morning.
- General fatigue, loss of appetite and possibly suffering from anemia.
- Inability to move in a smooth and stable manner.
- Elevation of body temperature and fever during the disease episodes.
- Drop in body weight.
- Rheumatoid nodules: These firm bumps of tissue under the skin most commonly form around pressure points, such as the elbows. However, these nodules can form anywhere in the body, including the lungs.

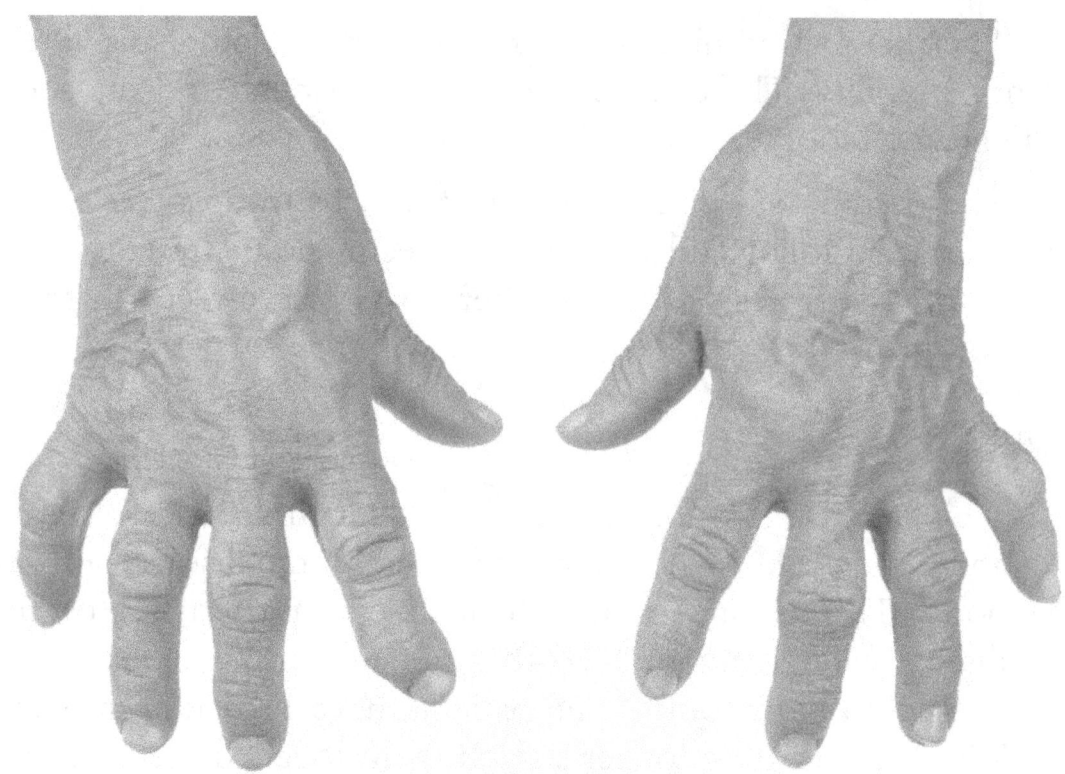

Effect of rheumatoid on hands

Complications

- With passage of time, erosion of the bone of the affected joint. The resulting inflammation thickens the synovium, which can eventually destroy the cartilage and bone within the joint. The tendons and ligaments that hold the joint together weaken and stretch. Gradually, the joint loses its shape and alignment.
- Dry eyes and mouth. People who have rheumatoid arthritis are much more likely to experience Sjogren's syndrome, a disorder that decreases the amount of moisture in your eyes and mouth.
- Infections. The disease itself and many of the medications used to combat rheumatoid arthritis can impair the immune system, leading to increased infections.
- Abnormal body composition. The proportion of fat to lean mass is often higher in people who have rheumatoid arthritis, even in people who have a normal body mass index (BMI).
- Carpal tunnel syndrome. If rheumatoid arthritis affects your wrists, the inflammation can compress the nerve that serves most of your hand and fingers.

- Heart problems. Rheumatoid arthritis can increase your risk of hardened and blocked arteries, as well as inflammation of the pericardium; the sac that encloses your heart to allow its movement without friction.
- Lung disease. People with rheumatoid arthritis have an increased risk of inflammation of the pleura that surrounds the lungs and scarring of the lung tissues, which can lead to progressive shortness of breath.
- Skin redness.
- Inflammation of Vasculitis.

Important Lab Tests

- Test of the Rheumatoid Factor (RF): Abnormal antibodies can be found in the blood of people with rheumatoid arthritis with simple blood testing. An antibody called "rheumatoid factor" (RF) can be found in 80% of patients with rheumatoid arthritis. RF test is a test to reveal the acquisition of the rheumatoid disease. The results are 70% to 90% correct. Patients with rheumatoid arthritis and rheumatoid factor are referred to as having "seropositive rheumatoid arthritis." Patients who are felt to have rheumatoid arthritis and do not have positive rheumatoid factor testing are referred to as having "seronegative rheumatoid arthritis."
- Sedimentation rate test (Sed rate): Sed rate is a crude measure of the inflammation of the joints. The sed rate actually measures how fast red blood cells fall to the bottom of a test tube. The sed rate is usually faster (high) during disease flares and slower (low) during remissions. a follow up test on the activity of the disease.
- Polymerase chain reaction (PCR): PCR to test C-reactive protein. Generally, PCR is a method widely used to rapidly make millions to billions of copies of a specific DNA sample, allowing scientists to take a very small sample of DNA and amplify it to a large enough amount to study in detail.
- Another blood test that is used to measure the degree of inflammation present in the body is the C-reactive protein. Blood testing may also reveal anemia, since anemia is common in rheumatoid arthritis, particularly because of the chronic inflammation.

The rheumatoid tests can also be abnormal in other systemic autoimmune and inflammatory medical conditions. Therefore, abnormalities in these blood tests alone are not sufficient for a firm diagnosis of rheumatoid arthritis.

Treatment

The treatment of the rheumatoid disease is aimed at cessation of the further development of the disease by administration of antiinflammation drugs, cortisone drugs are important. Nonsteroidal anti-inflammatory drugs (NSAIDs) may be also used. Such treatments have harmful side effects such as ulcers and stomach inflammation. This would require prescriptions for protection against such effects. This is in addition to the frequent change of the doses. Accordingly, the treatment must be under observation by a physician.

WHEN DOES THE CHANCE OF CONCEIVING A CHILD WITH DOWN SYNDROM INCREASE?

What is Down Syndrome?

Medically, a "syndrome" refers to a set of symptoms and distinctive medical signs which are correlated with each other and often associated with a particular disease or disorder. All or most of which must be present to diagnose the situation.

The word "Down" in is named after John Langdon Haydon Down, a British physician best known for his description of the genetic condition now known as the Down syndrome. The Down syndrome is a common chromosome disorder due to an extra chromosome number 21 (trisomy 21). Down syndrome causes mental retardation, a characteristic face, and multiple malformations. Down syndrome is a relatively common birth defect.

Due to his perception that children with Down syndrome shared facial similarities with those of Mongolian race the child diagnosed with was called mongoloid.

Symptoms and Signs

The symptoms and signs are related to the body shape and the cognitive aspects. Accordingly, it is easy to distinguish a child with merely by his/her features and bodily looks.

The important symptoms and signs are:

- The distinct shape of the head and face: generally small flat head, flat face, short neck, increased skin on back of neck, small and abnormal outer ears, protruding tongue, proportionally large tongue, slanted eyes (almond shape), abnormal teeth, flattened snub nose and a flat nasal bridge, Strabismus (abnormal alignment of the eyes; the condition of having a squint) and the presence of white spots in the iris called Brushfield spots.
- Stunted growth and short stature
- Shortened and wide hands and bent fifth fingertip.
- Single transverse palmar crease, normally the palm has three creases.
- Small feet and separation of first and second toes
- Narrow roof of mouth

- Undescended testicles.
- Flexible ligaments, low muscle tone (weak and limp muscles) which result in inability to carry loads and cope with physical work.

As of cognitive and mental symptoms and signs, the child is characterized by:

- Mental impairment
- Slowness in learning
- Slow developmental ability to talk
- Needs help in pronunciation of words
- Difficulty in concentration.

Health Problems

- Propensity to contract diseases, such as:
- Thyroid difficulties.
- Leukemia
- Seizure disorder
- Congenital heart disease
- Umbilical hernia
- Obstructive sleep apnea.

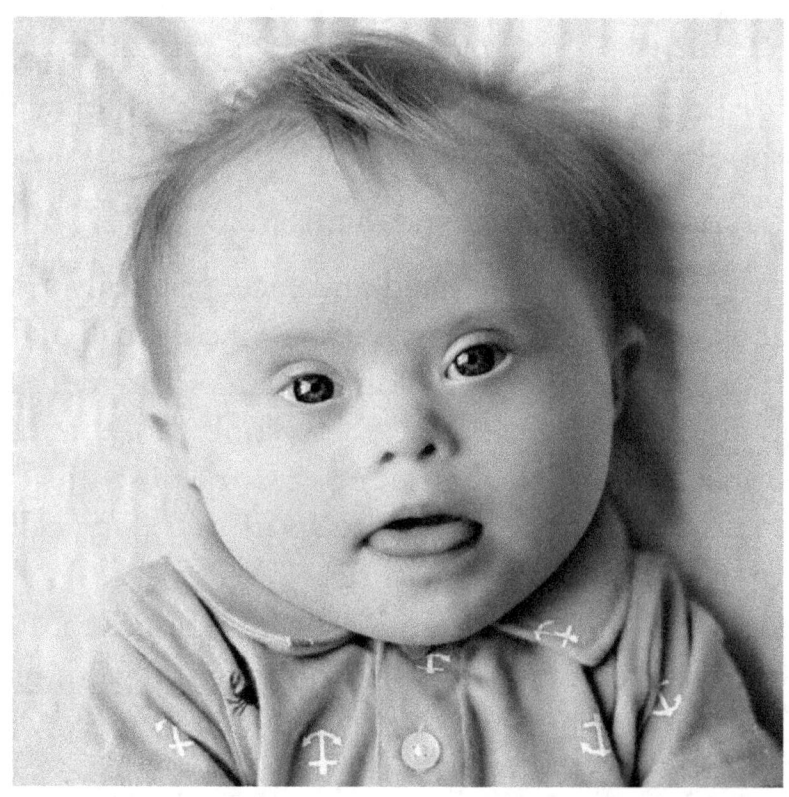

Child with Down syndrome

Causes of Down Syndrome

What do Chromosomes Mean?

Down syndrome is a common hereditary disease connected with chromosomes and does not transfer through genes.

The chromosomes are bodies that look like strings and formed from DNA and protein. They are present in the body cells and can be seen under a light microscope. They carry hereditary information about the human being through the genes. The number of chromosomes in human are 46 in each cell; 23 are inherited from the father and 23 from the mother during the genetic formation.

In the case of the Down syndrome, there is a defect in the chromosomes in the body of the fetus wherein there is a third replica whether complete or short in the chromosome number 21. Accordingly, the total number of chromosomes is 47 instead of 46. This situation is called Trisomy 21, that is the outcome of a defect in the division of the cells.

The fetus carries an extra inherited matter than normal which causes distinct changes in the baby with Down syndrome.

We do not know the reason for the difference in the chromosome. Nevertheless, it can be noticed that the likelihood of giving birth to a child with Down syndrome increases with the age of the mother giving birth. It was found that the likelihood of giving birth to a child with Down syndrome by a 40 years mother is 9 times that of a mother 30 years old. Furthermore, the birth of a child with Down syndrome in a family increases the chance of having another child having the same problem.

The diagnosis of the Down syndrome before giving birth is possible. Accordingly, it is advisable for a mother at an age over 35 years to examine the fetus before birth by a specialist to detect the status of the unborn. If the unborn has the Down syndrome abortion is advisable.

Treatment

There is no treatment to the Down syndrome. However, it is possible to treat some of the associated health problems, such as the heart problems, physical therapy to overcome muscles weakness. This in addition to speech therapy to improve the child's speech.

WHAT ARE THE CHANCES OF ACQUISITION OF BREAST CANCER?

Potential Causes

Breast cancer is known to be contracted by some women. Nevertheless, it is not a common knowledge that it can be acquired by men as well, although it is rare.

Accordingly, the gender is one of the factors that increase the likelihood of contracting the disease in addition to other factors, such as:

Hereditary Factor:

It is possible that a Genetic Mutation may take place leading to changes in specific genes, such as BRCA 1 or BRCA 2 in a manner that result in breast cancer. The daughters inherit such defective gene from their parents. However, the occurrence of such hereditary cancer is limited to 5% to 10% only.

Sometimes there is hereditary inclination to contract the disease without inheriting the genes among family members.

The chance for infection by breast cancer of a mother who got the disease before she reached 50 years of age increases by 1.6% if the mother contracted the disease after the mother passed the 50 years of age.

The Estrogen Hormone:

The estrogen hormone has a strong connection with the breast cancer. Estrogen is present in the body of females until menopause; that is when the ovary stops producing the hormone.

However, the increased exposure to estrogen can be a factor that aids in getting the disease, such as in the following cases:

- Early puberty.
- Late menopause.
- The resort to administration of synthetic estrogen as a substitute to reduce the problems associated with the menopause.
- Use of birth control pills.
- Obesity: As the fat accumulation in the body increases the exposure of the body to the estrogen since it is produced and stored in the

fatty cells. Accordingly, the obese female is likely to have breast cancer than the slim one after menopause.

Breast Cancer in one Breast

In case one breast only has the cancer, there is an increasing chance for the other breast contract cancer. In this case medications promoting protection are necessary.

Having no Children or no Breast Feeding:

Children delivery and breast-feeding cause physiological hormone changes which benefit the mother. This is why the breast cancer is more prevalent among nuns.

The Density of the Breast Tissues

The denser the breast tissues are the higher the probability of acquiring breast cancer. The probability increase can reach up to about 10%. This is since the higher density is associated with higher presence of estrogen. When the breast tissue is dense, the breast cancer sometimes does not appear in the mammogram at the beginning and it is discovered at a later stage.

Other Factors

- Fibrocystic Breast Disease
- Increase Exposure to Radiation
- Excessive Smoking
- Alcohol Drinking.

Symptoms

Self-diagnosis of the two breast is absolutely important. It relies on the comparison between the two breasts in terms of shape. The palpation (a method of feeling with the fingers or hands during a physical examination) may lead to discovery symptoms indicative of possible contraction of the disease, such as:

- Change in volume, shape, projection or looks of any of the two breasts (naturally the two breasts may slightly differ in size from one another)
- Change in the position of the nipples, upward direction.

- Appearance of secretion from the nipple for an unexplained reason.
- Feeling a lump in the breast tissue without feeling pain.
- Localized discoloration of the skin, the color is like the color of an orange rind.
- When lifting the arms up; in front of a mirror, one of the breasts fail to response to motion relative to the other.

What are the Expected Repercussions?

Early discovery of breast cancer prevents any adverse conditions and make the recovery more probable. The delay in discovery may cause the cancerous cells to spread in the lymphatic glands under the arm next to the affected breast. After that, the cancerous cells may move in the blood stream. The body becomes open and the cancerous cells can reach different organs.

Diagnosis and Treatment

The outcome of the self-examination can be verified by mammography, biopsy or enucleating the growth and testing it.

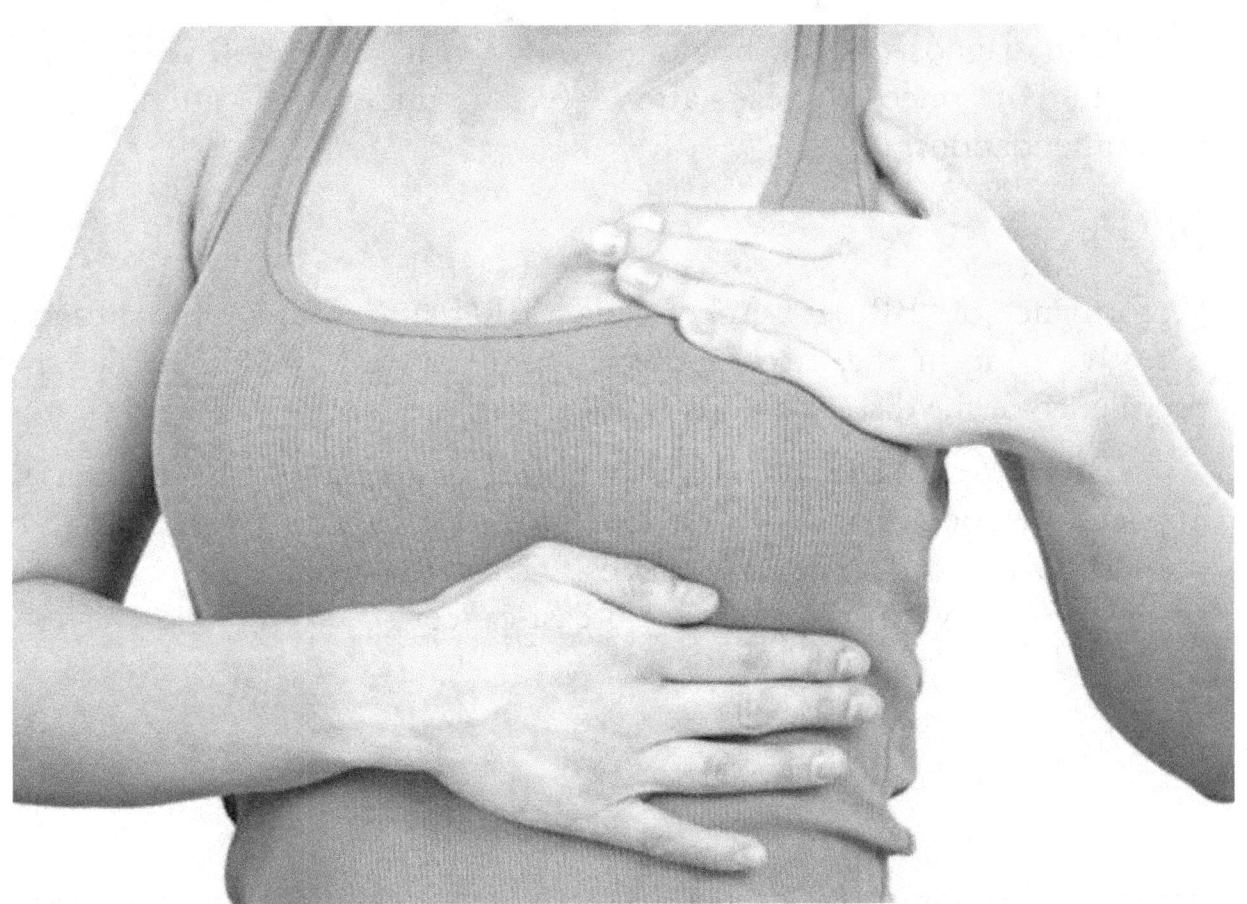

Change one breast compared to the other in self-diagnosis

The treatment of breast cancer is dependent of the stage of the spread of the disease. However, in all cases the tumor or the whole breast have to be removed, Furthermore, the lymphatic glands under the arm next to the affected breast has to be examined and possibly enucleated.

This may be followed by chemotherapy or radiotherapy.

Prevention

Self-Diagnosis:

Routine performance of the test to check any changes in the breast shape or tissues. It is preferred that the test be performed after a few days from the menstruation period, since the menstruation causes changes in the breasts including enlargement.

Mammography:

Mammography is necessary especially when breast cancer is prevalent in the family or in the case of propensity to infection for other reasons.

The diagnosis has to be done every 3 years before 40 years of age and at the rate of once a year after 40, or under the attending physician recommendations.

BRCA

Performance of "BReast CAncer gene" (BRCA) to examine the presence of any defective gene in the case of the existence of any hereditary factor and the prevalence of the disease among members of the family.

BRCA1 and BRCA2 are two different genes that have been found to impact a person's chances of developing breast cancer. Every human has both the BRCA1 and BRCA2 genes. Despite what their names might suggest, BRCA genes do not cause breast cancer.

SPLIT OF THE AORTA, IS IT RELATED TO A HERIDETATY DEFECT

Dissection Case

I have a friend who was on a tourism trip to Italy. When he was in his way back to the hotel, he was taken by surprise without any prewarning as he felt an agonizing pain in his chest wherein, he seemed to have something being torn apart inside. He fell on the ground squirming, as if he were a heroin addict and is suffering from a state of withdrawal. This made the people around hesitant to come close to him.

Performing an echocardiogram and taking images of the heart and the aorta showed a dissection in the aorta and a reverberation in the valve of the aorta.

This was the second time that the same thing has taken place in the family years before. His brother passed by the same heart condition when he was in same age of 50.

Aorta

The aorta looks like the main water pipe in a house wherein it distributes the water to other smaller pipes so that the water can reach different site in the house.

The blood goes from the heart to the aorta for distribution all over the body through smaller and smaller veins. The wall of the aorta is made of three layers; namely:

- Adventitia the outermost layer of the wall of a blood vessel and is formed of connective tissues, Collagen, and flexible fibers that allow the veins to expand.
- The tunica media (middle coat) or media for short, is the middle layer (tunica) of an artery or vein. It lies between the intima on the inside and the tunica externa on the outside. Tunica media is made up of smooth muscle cells, elastic tissue and collagen. It is the thickest layer.
- Intima is the internal layer and is smooth with elastic tissue through which the blood flows.

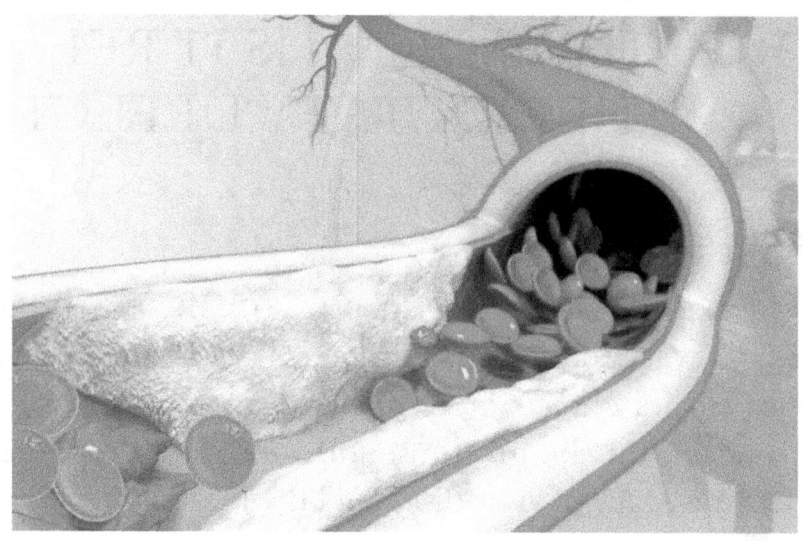

Layers of the aorta

The aorta artery comprises three parts:

- The thoracic aorta or ascending aorta extends from the aorta valve and ascends upward in the chest.
- The aortic arch from which a multitude of arteries branch out to distribute the blood to the upper parts of the body.
- Abdominal aorta or descending aorta to distribute the blood to the lower parts of the body and it is the largest part of the aorta.

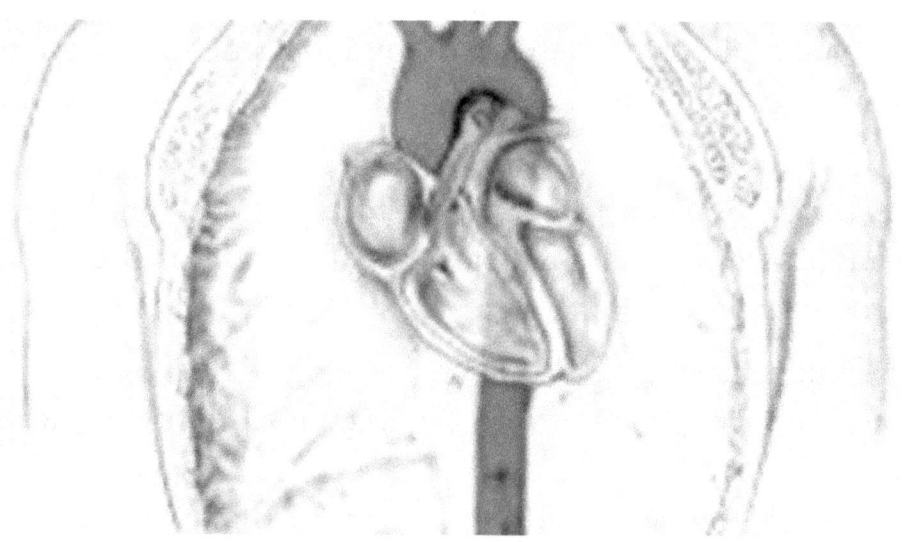

Aorta structure

What does the Aortic Dissection Mean?

In the case of the aortic dissection a sudden dissection or tear takes place in the intima through which the blood flows. According to that the blood flows through the next layer or media and less blood reaches the brains and the organs. This is a very serious situation. If it is not detected and surgically treated in an urgent matter the tear could increase and the arteries explode leading to death. Sometime a complete tear takes place and the artery explodes and death takes place without knowing the reason.

The dissection can occur in the ascending aorta, the aortic arch or the descending aorta. Sometimes the dissection take place in the three parts at the same time.

The symptoms are as follows:
- Excoriating pain in the chest which can reach the back in the case of dissection of the descending aorta.
- Drop in the blood pressure.
- Drop in the pulse rate.
- Pale face.
- General fatigue
- Severe pain in the stomach and a localized pulsation around the bellybutton in the case of dissection in the descending aorta.

The case is like the heart attack, nevertheless, it is more painful and devastating.

Strangely enough this case has relatively increase among the youth and may lead to sudden death.

Classification

The dissection may be classified as:
- Dissection of the ascending aorta with or without the aortic arch, Type A.
- Dissection of the descending aorta; Type B.

The dissection may be also classified as:
- Dissection of the ascending aorta in any place without the aortic arch, Type 1.
- Dissection of the ascending aorta with the aortic arch, Type 2.
- Dissection of the descending aorta; Type 3.

Why does the Dissection of the Aorta Occur?

- ❖ The dissection problem takes place among members of some families. Accordingly, it is called: Familial Aortic Dissection (FAD).
- ❖ There is no specific gene connected to the dissection case. Hence, it does not transfer by inheritance. However, one can say that there is a hereditary inclination to acquire the disease or it may result from recession of a specific gene; however, that postulate is not supported by evidence.
- ❖ Extreme elevation of blood pressure (this may take place because of the dissection)
- ❖ Hardening of the arteries (this may take place because of the dissection).
- ❖ Excess smoking may promote dissection.
- ❖ Weakness in the connective tissues. This is a hereditary defect as in the Marfan syndrome.

Treatment

In the case of dissection of the ascending aorta with the aortic arch (Type 2), the treatment involves replacement of the deteriorated part by a Dacron graft. If that is accompanied by dissection of the descending aorta; Type 3, the above surgery may be satisfactory since the performance of the descending aorta will be improved as the blood will flow down in a smooth natural way. The widened aorta valve may be replaced of modified,

Such surgery is rather very complicated and involves high risk due to increase in the fatality percentage and it requires an experienced surgeon specialized in such procedures.

It is customary to prescribe medications; especially of the beta blockers type, to maintain the blood pressure. Other medications may be prescribed from the astatines class to protect against precipitation of the cholesterol in the arteries.

HUNTINGTON DISEASE … IS THE INVOLUNTARY MUSCLE MOVEMENTS HERIDITARY?

The Victims of the Disease

I recall a young man who used to move his hands and fingers in the air in a motion that seemed involuntary. He moves erratically and his speech is muffled and hard to understand. During my studies in the medical school I got to know that the symptoms displayed by that young man are exactly those of a disease we were studying at the time, which is Huntington Disease. Through the practice of my profession, after graduation I encountered two cases suffering from that same disease, which was named after George Huntington, the first to describe the disease in the eighties of the nineteenth century.

What is the Defect that Promotes that Disease?

The defect that promotes the Huntington disease is in the presence of a defective gene on the chromosome number 4. That defect is associated with accumulation of a protein harmful to the brains and lead to the destruction of the nerve fibers in the basal ganglia. the basal ganglia is a group of structures linked to the thalamus in the base of the brain and involved in coordination of movement). This is accompanied by disturbance in the mental functions and the mood. The protein is called Huntington protein.

This disease is hereditary and is dominant. This means that the transfer from the father or the mother to their children increases the likelihood of contracting the disease.

What is the Potential of Contracting the Huntington Disease?

- The acquisition of the father or the mother to the defective gene leads to the transfer of the disease to their children with a probability of 50%. This increases to 75% if both parents have the defective gene. Nevertheless, the disease can be contracted by the whole family!
- There is no gender difference in contracting the disease; that is it can be equally contracted by males and females.

- ❖ The disease exists around the whole world and in different races, however, it is rare. Nevertheless, the disease occurs at a higher rate among Americans and Caucasians. In the US one in ten thousand are victims of the disease, which is relatively a high ratio. This is why an organization was founded for the disease in the USA. It is called: Huntington Disease Society of America (HDSA).
- ❖ Ordinarily the disease prevails in people between 30 and 50 years of age. However, it may affect may be contracted by teens. When contracted by people under 20 years of age it is called: Juvenile Huntington Disease.
- ❖ The disease may be acquired by a member of the family despite the notion that the parents being free from the defective gene. In this case, there are two possibilities. The first is that there is an error in the diagnosis of one of the parents, in spite of being affected by the person can be diagnosed as having Parkinson's Disease, which has similar symptoms to those of the Huntington disease. The second possibility is genetic mutation which has led to contracting the disease. The probability of such occurrence is not more than 10%.

Symptoms

The main symptom is the inability to control the movement and its involuntary and uncoordinated occurrence. This is called chorea (or choreia, occasionally) in the medical field. Chorea is an abnormal involuntary movement disorder, one of a group of neurological disorders called dyskinesias. The term chorea is derived from the Ancient Greek "dance", as the quick movements of the feet or hands are comparable to dancing.

Those involuntary movements can occur by different limbs as the arms, fingers, legs or the head.

It also takes place by the muscles of the face and eyes. Accordingly, the patient may stumble in his walk, may encounter difficulty in chewing food because of the messed-up muscles that move the jaws. Repetitious involuntary movements are referred to by some as the "hereditary dancer" disease.

Another symptom is the change in the mental processes such as the inability to concentrate and to learn as well as the lapses of memory. The patient oftentimes is unable to pronounce the word correctly or legibly.

The disease has great effect on the mood. Most likely the patient will suffer from depression and anxiety. Therefore, the patient usually tends to commit suicide. The great burden of the Huntington disease is likely to shorten the patient's life and end up dying at young age.

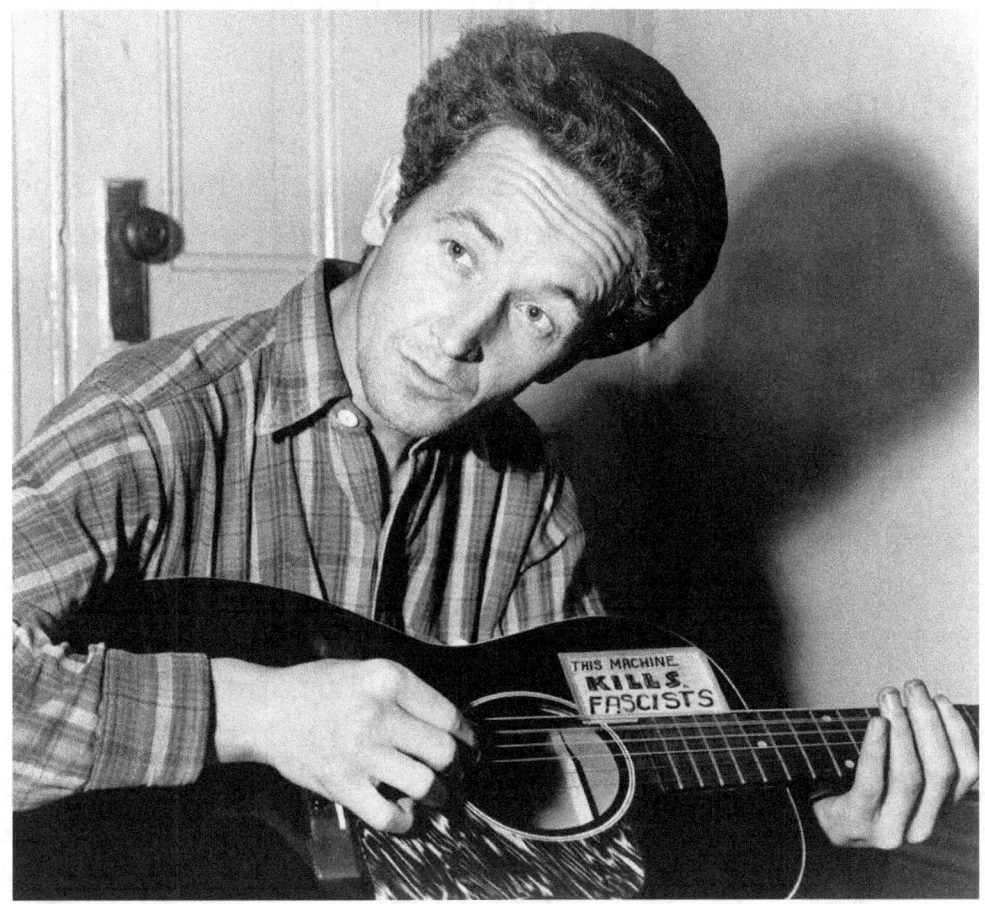

One of the most famous people who have Huntington Disease was the American singer Woody Guthrie, who died in 1967 at the age of 55 years

Diagnosis and Treatment

In addition to the aforementioned symptoms, the observations can be verified by performing Magnetic resonance imaging (MRI) or computerized tomography scan (CT or CAT scan) on the brains to detect the destruction of the nerve fibers in the basal ganglia. It is also possible to conduct a hereditary assessment to detect the defective gene which has been identified in 1993.

There is no treatment for the Huntington disease. However, the symptoms can be alleviated by prescription of psychological and nerve drugs. Some of the recent medications may enable the patient to control the disease progress.

WHY SOME PEOPLE ARE BALD AND OTHERS ARE NOT?

Hair Factory

The hair factory is the hair follicles in the scalp, which does not seize working on the replacement of lost hair by new hair through a hair growth cycle. the performance of the hair follicles is affected by age. As the person gets older, they get lazy and subsequently the rate of falling hair exceeds the rate of growth of new hair. The density of her thins with progress in age.

The Naughty Hormone!

The hair follicles are most affected by the male hormone, testosterone or more precisely its the hormone version Dihydroxytestosterone (DHT). About 10% of the testosterone converts into DHT in the testicles and prostate with the action of the enzyme 5-Alpha-Reductase. This DHT form of the testosterone is much stronger since it connects to the same cell receptors of the testosterone. The receptors are proteins that allow or block matter that desires to get into the cell. The DHT and the testosterone are androgens; that is the material that constructs the male features such as the muscle strength. Therefore, the receptors of the DHT and the testosterone are called androgen receptors (AR).

The question here is why this version of the testosterone harmful or troublesome hormones?

This is because the DHT hormone is not only connected to boldness but also to the benign enlargement of the prostate as well as promotion of prostate cancer. This does not mean that the presence of the DHR always leads to trouble!

What is the DHT Connection to Hereditary Baldness?

One may notice that baldness progresses in some families than others. Baldness may start very early in some families; that is around the ages between twenties and thirties. It was found that this phenomenon is hereditary or more precisely related to the gene connected to the Androgen Receptors Gene (AR Gene).

That AR gene makes the AR more sensitive to the DHT hormone or it increases their number. That gene is also connected to the increase of DHT above the normal level, which depends on the heredity aspects. In all cases, with the increase in DHT the hair follicles become lethargic, unable to produce new hair and their life is shortened.

This is why there is a bald person and another who isn't!

Do Women Get Bald?

One may wonder to learn that the testosterone hormones are present in females. Furthermore, it is the testosterone which is responsible for the female sex drive. Nevertheless, testosterone in females is limited compared to men.

Accordingly, women are subject to the hereditary baldness but at a less extent than men.

Is the Baldness Gene Hereditary?

Yes, children inherit the AR gene from their parents. Therefore, all the children or some of them are expected to grow bald at certain age; similar to the age at which their parents became bald.

The Form of Hereditary Baldness

Normally Male Pattern Alopecia starts at the temples and the hairline gradually recedes such as the remaining hair appears in the form of the cap letter M or it starts at the crown of the head. The baldness may continue to stretch until the whole hair disappears.

With female pattern baldness, thinning occurs on the top and crown of the head. This thinning in women often starts as a widening of the center hair part that leaves the front hairline unaffected.

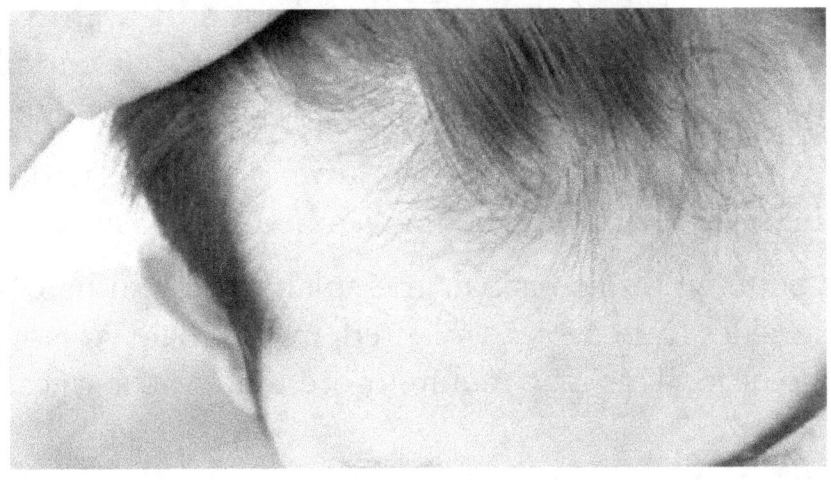

Baldness at the upper side of the head and recessed hairline

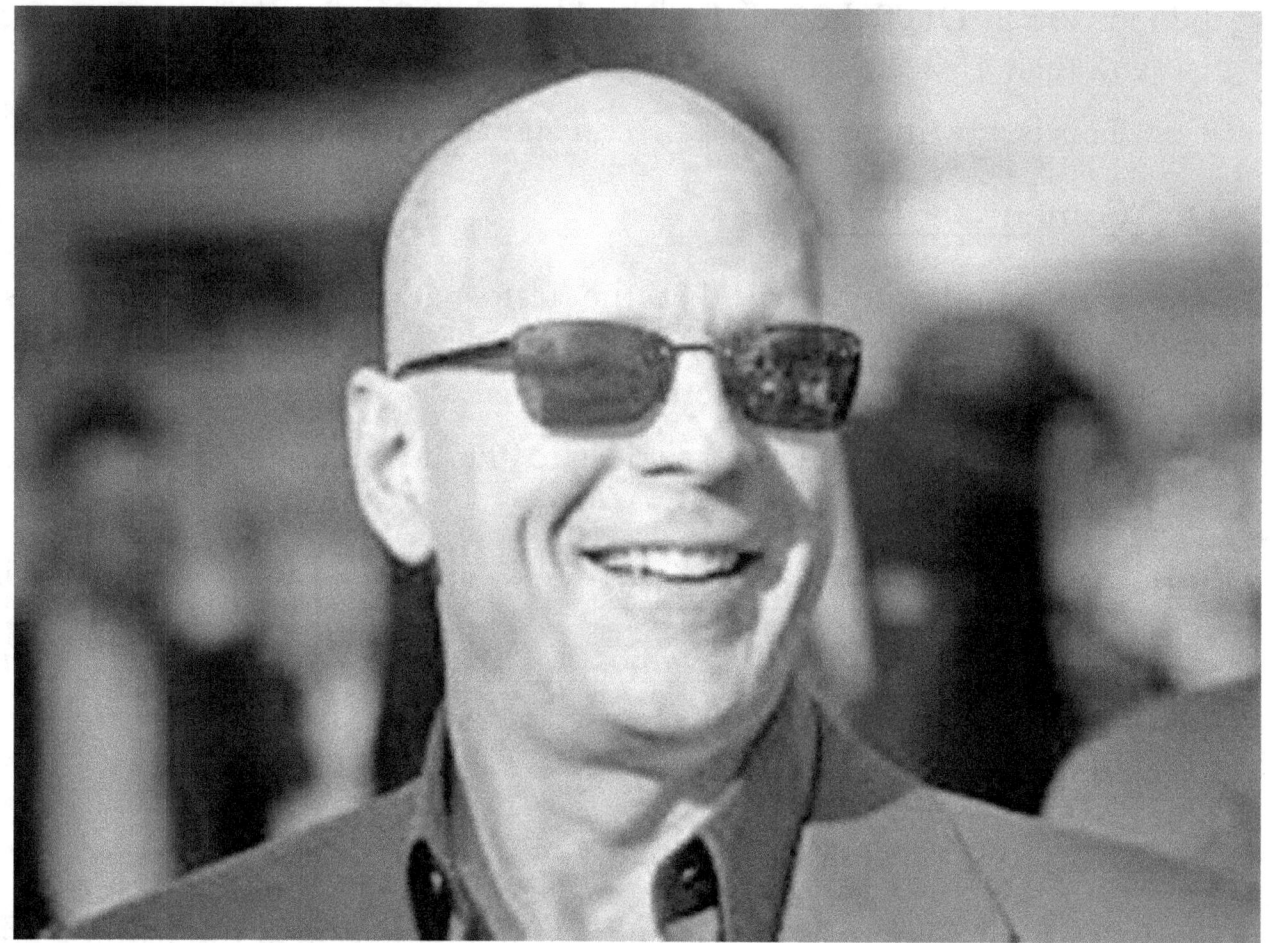

Bruce Willis, a famous American actor who is totally bald

How can Baldness be Treated?

Since baldness is connected to the hormone DHT, the baldness can be treated by an antihormone drug. Such drug is available. Nonetheless, one cannot expect that the hair will grow to the full extent before boldness. The drug will help slight thin growth of the hair over a long period of use. In addition to this type of medication, alternatively one may use a drug that curtail the production of DHT. Even in this case one might not hope that the baldness will disappear.

There are other treatments that are not drug related, such as injection of plasma in the scalp. Such treatment gives better outcome.

Yet a better approach is hair transplant, wherein hair from the back of the scalp or the sides can be transplanted in the bald areas in the front or the middle of the head. This may require more than one surgical procedure.

There are also attempts to use stem cells in rejuvenation of the hair follicles.

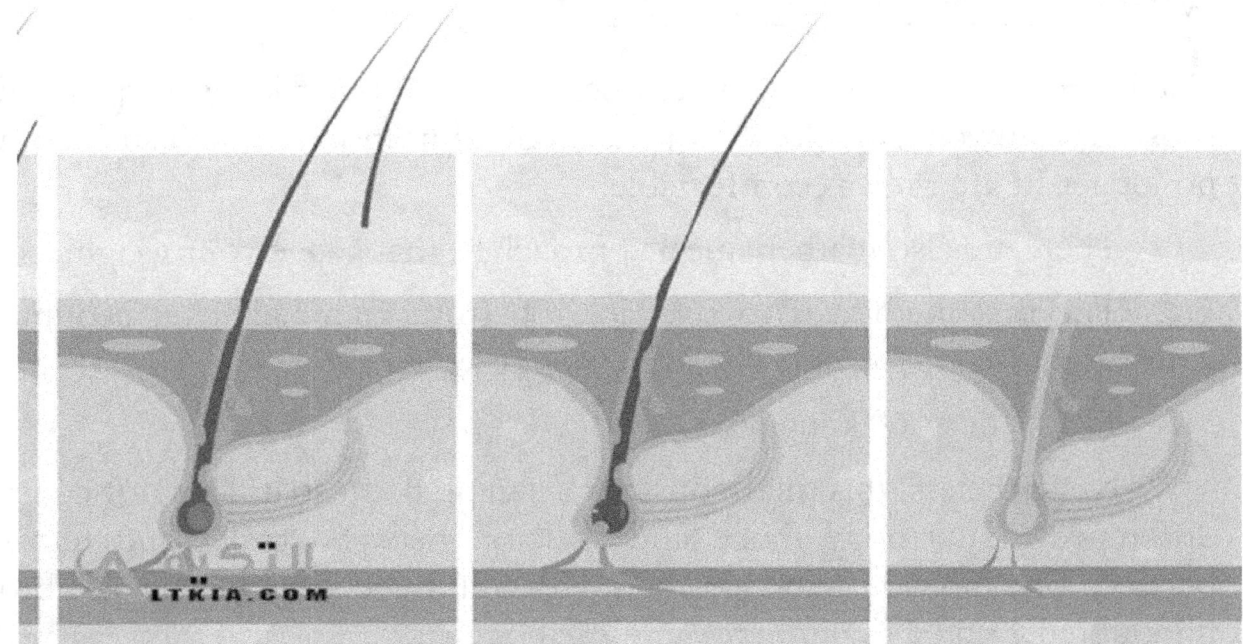

Hair Follicle a part inside the hair wherein hair grow upward

IS OBESITY HEREDITARY?

When Can You Say You are Fat?

The mirror can tell you if you are obese or not. Your friends, acquaintance and those around you can tell. A more accurate indication are the usual clothes that no longer fit after it was comfortable.

There are also mathematical approaches, that gauge your weight, such as:

The first method is to subtract 100 from your height in centimeters. If your height is say, 160 cm. The ideal weight would be:

160 – 100 = 60 kilogram

Nevertheless, this method is not accurate because it does not consider the difference in the body frame and skeleton between males and females and between one individual and another. The with huge skeleton big and broad will undoubtedly find a slight increase in their weight.

The more precise way is in using the Body Mass Index (BMI), which represents the relationship between height and weight. This is also the standard method approved by the WHO and NIH.

This method is based on the quotient of the body weight in kilogram and the square of the height in meters.

For example, using the International System of Units (SI):

If the weight is 70 kilograms, the height is 175 cm or 1.75 m, the result will be:

$70 \div (1.75)^2 \approx 22.9$

The results are analyzed as follows:

Light obesity: 30-35

Medium obesity: 35-40

Extreme obesity: ≥ 40.

Using the US National System of Units:

BMI = {weight, lbs./{(height, in.)^2} × 703

Example: Weight = 180 lb.; height = 68 in.

BMI = 180/{(68)^2} × 703 = 27.5

The Role of Inheritance

- ❖ Clearly the obesity is hereditary, or to less extent the inclination to get weight is more prevalent in some families than others.
- ❖ There is no specific gene connected to obesity. However, obesity relates to a gamut of genetic factors.
- ❖ Most of the obesity cases relate to the lifestyle, such as eating in excess, inclination to eat high calories food, inactivity. The hereditary obesity is limited in general. Its percentage differ from one society to another. It may reach more than 5%.
- ❖ When the parents are extremely obese, the obesity of their children may reach 80%, while it may reach to about 7% or less if the parents have moderate weight.
- ❖ Some studies revealed that if an Identical Twin are obese, they will be obese in the same way which shows that inheritance plays a factor since their genes are exactly the same.
- ❖ Some individuals have a hereditary propensity for fat accumulation more than fat consumption which increases the likelihood of getting fat.
- ❖ Inheritance plays a role in how fat is distributed in the body, such as storing the fat in the buttock more than anywhere else.
- ❖ Obesity is connected to the number of fat cells a person had at birth. The number stays the same. The more the number the higher the potential of being fat as a baby as well as later on. However, in some other cases the number of fat cells is average, but the fat cells are elastic or large in size. In this case the cells have the capacity to store excess fat which leads to obesity. In both cases, the reduction of the excess weight can be relatively high.
- ❖ Fat cells produce and store fat. They are naturally renewed at a rate of 10% per year. This is in addition to the fat that we get from food and which is stored in the adipose tissue under the skin and between the different organs, such as around the intestines and heart as soft cushions for protection. We also benefit from these fats as a source of energy and for maintaining the body temperature.
- ❖ The excess in fat cells relate to the thickness of the adipose tissue under the skin by hereditary factors.

Increase of the number of fat cells in childhood increase the potential of being obese after puberty by three times compared to those with ordinary fat cells.

The body is capable of construction of new fat cells in the case of absolute necessity as is in the case of a surgery to obliterate part of the adipose tissue or sucking large amounts of fat. Accordingly, it is necessary for those who resort to those surgeries to reduce weight or to modify the stature to follow a healthy diet appropriate for avoiding weight increase in the second round.

Leptin Hormone

The Leptin hormone is the hormone of satiety. It is produced by the fat cells from some type of protein, especially from the white fat tissues under the skin which work as the energy storage and surround the body to insulate it and maintain its temperature. This hormone has receptors in the brains in the hypothalamus. Through this nerve connection this hormone manages the body energy, limit the appetite to avoid excessive feeding.

It is believed that one of the causes of obesity is the resistance of the effect of the Leptin hormone and the subsequent overeating. The reason may be the ineffectiveness or shortage in its production. This may take place due to a fast increase in the related gene.

Since that hormone is connected with the appetite, its consumption in a synthesized form can play a role in treatment of obesity. Nevertheless, such idea is still under review and subject of controversy.

Finally, the presence of heredity factors in obesity does not eliminate the opportunity for weight reduction through management of the nutrition aspects, engagement in physical activities to consume the excess calories. Nonetheless, such undertaking requires additional efforts and time compared to the obesity cases which are not related to heredity factors.

BIPOLAR DISORDER ... DO WE INHERIT DEPRESSION AND MANIA EPISODES?

In the Psychiatry Ward

I still recall until now, the day is was in my tour in the psychological and neurological diseases wing at the hospital where I was an intern. I and my physician colleagues were taken by surprise. A girl in her twenties entered breaking into loud laughter and swinging gallantly in her walk. We were more or less shocked when she approached us to give us hugs. She was elated and did not stop talking crackling and moving from one subject to the next, dancing like having a trance.

That girl was a live model of mania.

Following a thorough diagnosis of her case she was admitted and placed in a private room under guard due to her aggressiveness and extreme lewd behavior, one of the symptoms of her case. The administration was worried she may leave the hospital pregnant.

That reminded me of another patient suffering from a case like hers who tried to sexually assault one of our colleagues, a female physician!

What is Meant by Bipolar Disorder?

Bipolar disorder is a type of mental disorder or psychosis that combines two opposite extremes: depression episodes and manic (merry and euphoric) episodes. Accordingly, it is referred to as Manic Depressive Psychosis.

The manic episode as in the case of the two patients; mentioned above, is distinguished by the following symptoms:

- The body of the patients acquire a high level of energy, so they go in a frenzy of restless commotions and motions. They hardly stop ranting, the thoughts rush in the brains as colliding storms, like a bird losing its campus jumping from one branch to another in what may be describes as "Flight of Ideas."
- Sexual arousal.
- Unusual euphoria that drives the patient to hysteric dancing and laughter.
- The high level of energy causes hyperactivity and insomnia.

- The behavior is not controlled by reasoning or deliberation which leads to taking undue risks without thinking of the consequences or repercussions.

In contrast, the depression mode is accompanied by exhaustion, and a state of withdrawal and miserable feelings wherein the symptoms include:

- Cessation of activities, lack of interest in life as a whole and inability to enjoy what used to be joyful before.
- Loss of appetite.
- Regrets and guilty feelings and tendency to self-blame.
- Restless sleep, frequent wakening and early rising with no desire to get up.
- Pessimism and suicidal temptations.
- The urge to cry.

Such episodes are repetitive and occur at a rate that differs from on case to the other. The mania is relatively shorter than the depression and may not exceed couple of days. The depression is much longer and may exceed weeks or months if there is no treatment.

The episodes keep on alternating in a chronic manner. They may stop for long time and the patient feels normal. However, a relapse may take place, especially when the patient neglects prescribed treatments by physicians. This is actually what happens in many cases.

What is the Cause for the Disorder?

The disorder is triggered by a defect of the neurotransmitters in the brains that affect the mood, such as serotonin, dopamine and norepinephrine. The hereditary factors play an important role in this disorder. The environment and the family climate also play a role, such as the mistreatment and cruel treatment during childhood. Psychological treatments are successful in some cases.

The Hereditary Role

- There is no difference between the genders as the disorder occurs to females and males with almost the same percentage and it takes place usually in the twentieth and thirtieth of age.

- There is no clear difference among the offsprings. Nevertheless, in a study in the USA, it was shown that the disorder is more prevalent among those from European or African descent compare to those from Asian roots.
- Some statistics show that about 1% to 3% of the world population have suffered from such disorder in a stage of their life and 6.4% of the Americans suffer from some type of bipolar disorder.
- The disorder is inherited at a percentage of about 25%. If any of the parents suffers from the disorder it is likely the children will suffer too. Accordingly, the disorder is transferred in some families.
- A recessive gene may cause the disorder. In this case the disorder is not connected to the grandparents.
- Although the hereditary factor plays a role in that disorder, no chromosome or gene have been identified as the cause for the disorder.
- In a study of the disorder among twins, it was found that the occurrence of the disorder among identical twins; wherein the genes are identical, is about 40%. That is, the contracting the disorder by one of the twins does not necessitate the contracting by the other, although it is expected that both will suffer from the disorder at the same time. The percentage among non-identical twins is only 5%.

Diagnosis

There is no specific test to diagnose the disorder; however the imaging of the brains may help exclude other disease that are connected to physical brains problem.

Treatment

- The lithium treatment could benefit in the control of the episodes, reducing the frequency of the episodes, and in preventing the suicidal thoughts.
- The use of drugs for the psychosis during acute episodes.
- Treatment by electric shocks may be beneficial during acute depression.
- Psychiatric treatment.

Famous People having Bipolar Disorder

The American singer Rosemary Clooney suffered from the bipolar disorder. Also the famous Egyptian poet and cartoonist Salah Gahin suffered from bipolar disorder in a way that affected his work.

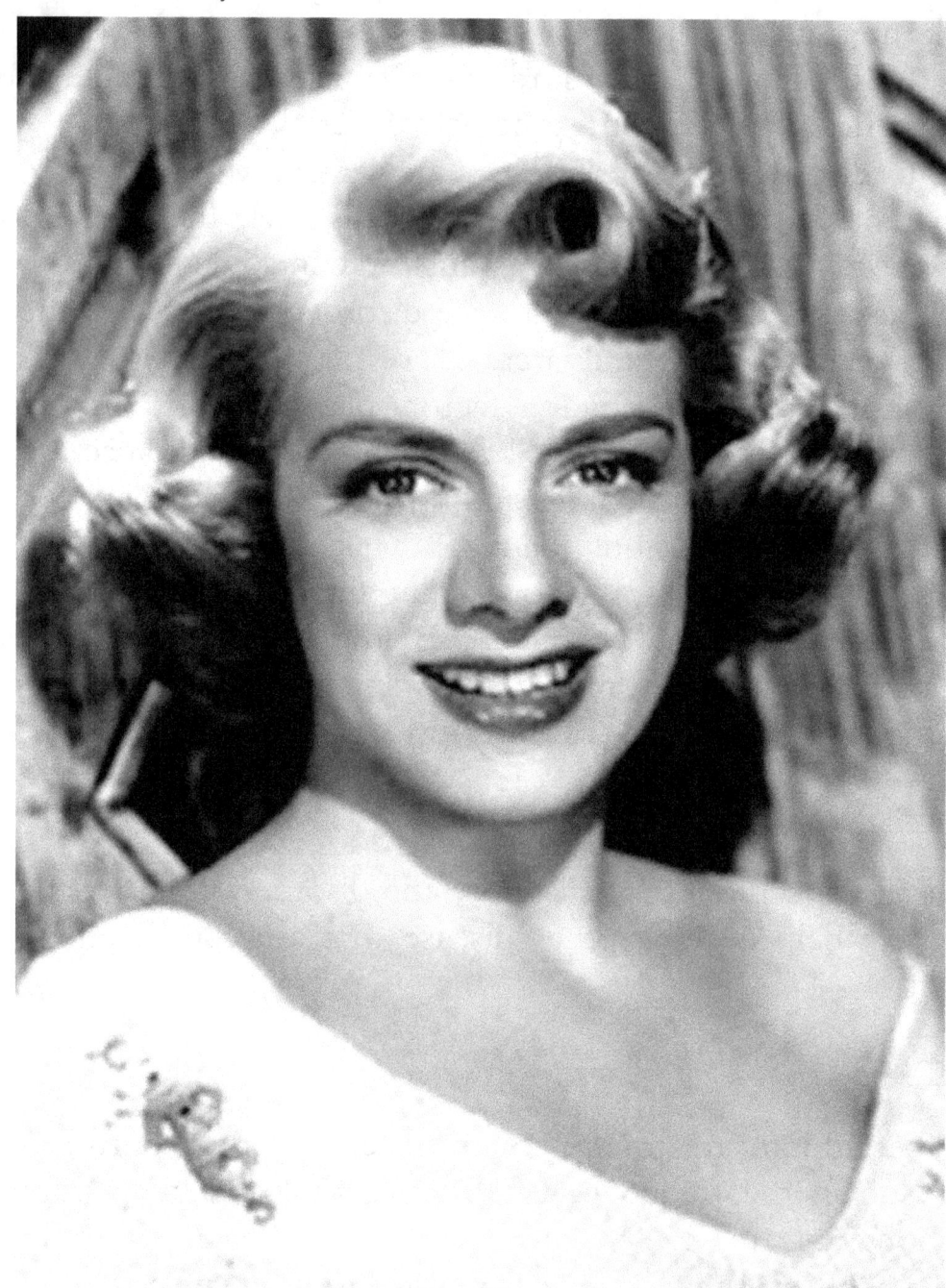

Rosemary Clooney

HEREDITARY MUSCULAR WEAKNESS (DUCHENNE MUSCULAR DYSTROPHY)

Male Only Disease!

Muscular Dystrophy or the extreme muscle weakness that reaches atrophy (the shrinking stage) is a group of diseases. The most known of such diseases and which represents 50% of the group is Duchenne Muscular Dystrophy (DMD). As a hereditary disease DMD is like hemophilia. It is a for men only disease; however, females carry the disease gene without being affected except in very rare situations and to a very lenient extent. Why?

DMD is connected to the chromosome X (X- Linked Disorder) which could be dominant or recessive. Since the male has one X chromosome and one Y chromosome; that is he has XY chromosomes, any defective gene in X causes the sickness of the male. This is while the female has two chromosomes of type X; that is, she is XX. any defective gene in one X does not qualify her to catch the disease since the presence of a healthy X will maintain her muscle strength.

What is the Cause of Muscle Weakness?

The DMD develops because of the unavailability of dystrophin; the protein necessary for building the muscles, maintaining their strength and tone. Such deficiency leads to reduction in the muscles' mass. This difficulty is connected to the presence of defective gene or a mutation of a gene. The DMD is a relatively rare disease, it affects 1 in 3,500 of males. In the USA the disease affects 200,000 yearly. It is worth mentioning that there is a society formed especially for the disease.

The DMD appears after a short time from birth; usually between 3 and 5 years old.

The Role of Inheritance

The DMD occurs in certain families wherein the children inherit the disease from one parent or both.

The effect of the mother carrying the gene is rather high. It was found that the mother who carries the defective gene passes it to her sons by a percentage of 50% and also passes it to her daughters by 50%. Nevertheless, the females only carry the defective gene and they do not contract the disease. However, they can pass it on to their sons when they have children.

The Muscles Affected by the Disease

Usually the muscle weakness is concentrated in the shoulders, the arms (without the hands), the thighs, the torso and the chest muscles. The chest affects the breathing. Accordingly, the patient suffers from breathing complications. The weakness extends to the heart muscle which gets enlarged and weakened. Such enlargement is not indication of strength but of cardiomyopathy. This is reason for the patient suffering from heart problems. Accordingly, most patients are subject to early death.

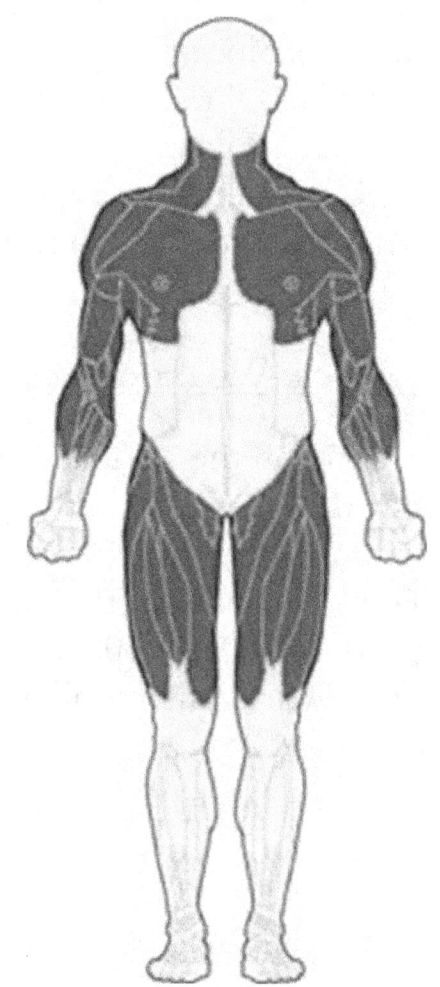

The muscles affected by the Duchenne disease

Symptoms

The mother can notice at an early stage that her baby has DMD, since the symptoms are:

- Difficulty in walking and the need for assistance,
- Slowness or wadding gait,
- Body imbalance when walking,
- Limited motion span,
- Hunch back or scoliosis.

How can this Disease be Diagnosed?

In addition to the symptoms and the DMD distinctive indication, the patient may need several tests such as:

- Electromyography of the muscles.
- Muscular Biopsy: in this case there is a distinct presence of the enzymes Creatine PhosphoKinase (CPK).

Treatment

- There is no treatment per se. However, there is trials of gene therapy.
- Use of steroids with the aim to stop the creeping muscle weakness.
- Physical therapy.
- Surgery may be done to straighten the bones connected to the weak muscles.

DOES PARKINSON DISEASE PREVAIL IN FAMILIES?

The Most Famous victims of Parkinson Disease

When the Parkinson's Disease (PD); which is also called the quivering paralysis is mentioned, one immediately recalls the American box champion Mohamed Ali who was infected by the disease when he was 38 years old. The disease turned him from and athlete to a person moving at low pace with continuous tremors.

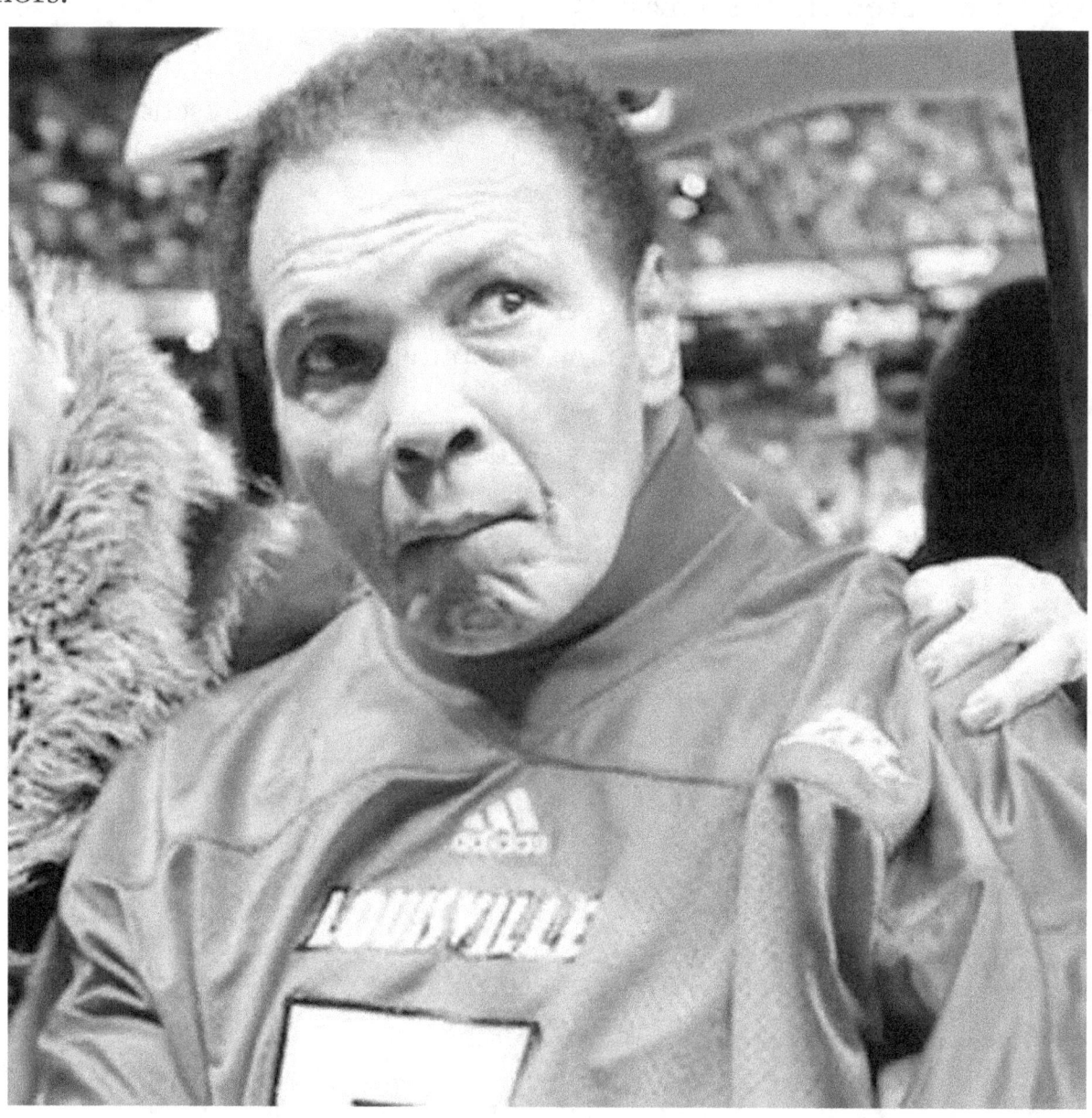

Mohamed Ali after Parkinson disease

Change in Brains Activity

The radical change that the PD does to the active life and muscular strength of the patient; as in the case of Mohamed Ali, results from deficiency in dopamine the nerve transmitter from the damage of the nerve cells that produce it in the brains. Following that major unnatural changes take place in the activities of the brains, which leads to the symptoms of the disease.

What is the Reason?

The reasons for acquiring the PD are not clear, however there are some plausible reasons, such as: frequent beating on the head (as was the case with Mohamed Ali) and exposure to pesticides and/or herbicides.

Hereditary Role

Inheritance plays a role in contracting PD, in some cases. Accordingly, there is a mix between the environmental and heredity factors that trigger the case.

- Gender: PD is a male thing to a great extent. Seldom one can find a female suffering from this disease.
- Age: PD occurs in the middle age; however usually affect elderly people after the age of 60.
- Race: In the US, the PD is more prevalent among Americans of African and Asian origin compared to white Americans. According to some statistics the number of PD victims is two hundred thousand yearly.
- Inheritance: The PD spread among specific families more than others. About 15% of the patients are from families wherein some kin suffered from PD; such as the father, the mother or a brother.
- Gene: The PD is connected to more than one gene. In about 5% of the cases, the disease takes place due to recession of the gene GBA1; however, this gene is non familial. Also, a recession may occur to the gene LRAK2 which is familial.

Symptoms

The PD starts in a slow gradual fashion and primarily affect the motor, however, that can be accompanied by non-motor movements.

- ❖ Motion: The patient movement during walking are slow and heavy; Bradykinesia, accompanied by stiffness, narrow movement span, and short paces. The patient may drag his feet as he walks. Sometimes he takes a sequence of fast paces that make him prone to fall on his face. The shuffling gait is a distinct symptom of PD. This makes the patient unable to have a good control on his balance and make him susceptible to tipping over and fall.
- ❖ Tremor: Tremors are also distinct symptoms of PD. Tremors start in the fingers of one hand and takes the form of rubbing the thumb by the forefinger as if he is counting banknotes. The tremor is distinguished by taking place during rest periods; that is the tremor stops if he held something be his fingers. The tremor can be in the head as if the patient is nodding. The patient is incapable of writing by hand due to the slowness of the motion combined with the tremor.
- ❖ Face: Lack of expression on the patient's face which looks as if he has a mask face.
- ❖ Speech: The patient's ability to talk is impaired and his speech is usually monotonous and slurred.
- ❖ Feeding: The patient may have difficulty chewing and swallowing because of the PD on the muscles involved in the eating process.

In addition to the movement-dependent symptoms there is other symptoms, such as: apathy, depression, constipation, amnesia, and hyposmia. A person with PD does not have to display all those symptoms. However the walking and the tremors are the main symbols.

Treatment

Parkinson disease is a chronic disease wherein all those who have it worldwide are treated by one drug, Levodopa to alleviate the symptoms related to the movement and the tremor. The medicine is absorbed in the intestine and transferred to the brains to convert into dopamine and thus reduce its deficiency.

There are also trials of gene therapy to correct the genetic defect associated with the PD.

HEREDITARY FAVA BEANS ANEMIA

The Strange Enzyme

The red blood cells produce the enzyme: Glucose-6-phosphate dehydrogenase (G6PD). That enzyme is necessary for the safety of the red blood cells since it protects them through chemical processes from oxidative damage and prevents their destruction at an early stage; that is before 120 days, the presumed lifetime.

The deficiency in the G6PD enzyme leads to destruction and defection in the red cells before the onset of anemia and the inability of the sufficient oxygen to reach the body cells. That is in addition to contracting jaundice which leads to yellowing of the skin and the whites of the eyes due to the loss of hemoglobin from the blood and its conversion to the yellow bilirubin matter.

The fava beans anemia is hereditary and commences to appear when the child starts to feed with the family. This usually happens after six months from birth or throughout the first years of the child's age.

The severity of the disease depends on the deficiency level of the G6PD enzyme. They range from light, medium and severe in which case the consequences are alarming and frequent blood transfusion is necessary.

What is the Relationship between Fava Beans and Anemia?!

The absence or deficiency in the G6PD enzyme can cause oxidative damage to the red blood cells before the presumed end of life. Such oxidization process is connected to specific food or medications and it is connected as well with infections such as a severe case of cold.

On the top of the food stuff is the legumes such as fava beans, English green fava beans (broad beans), peanuts and generally the beans which have two halves.

This is why the disease is referred to as favism in reference to the body reaction in the form of anemia to eating fava beans.

As of the medications and drugs that are connected to the anemia attacks. They include antimalarial medicines, sulfa drugs, chloramphenicol and some pain medications such as aspirin.

It is of the outmost importance for the mother of the affected child to keep the attending physician abreast of the status of her child and confirm his case of acquiring the fava beans anemia.

This anemia attacks suddenly without any prewarning. It can be discovered by mere chance after consumption of a quantity of fava beans (or similar legumes).

This reminds me of the first case I have encountered of the fava beans anemia, while I was an intern in the children hospital. A woman came to the hospital carrying her little child in a panic. She was scared about the welfare of her child who was about two years old. She indicated that his face is turning yellow and had hard time breathing. As I checked his medical history, I discovered that the symptoms showed up after having a meal of fava beans with his mother. That was the first time the mother got to know that her child acquired the fava beans anemia.

Symptoms

The mother may notice the following symptoms on her child after consuming a meal of a large quantity of fava beans: panting and shortness of breath, racing pulses, yellowing of the skin and the eye whites, pale face, stomach pain and the urine is dark in color and may be mixed with red color in case of seeping blood with the urine. This is in addition to slowness in the child growth in time.

Such symptoms may be followed be repercussions in severe cases. These include enlargement of the spleen wherein the deteriorated and broken red blood cells get accumulated. This may be accompanied by severe kidney inflammation.

However, in most cases the symptoms triggered by eating fava beans disappear after the passage of a few days without treatment.

How to Verify the Diagnostics of the Fava Beans Anemia?

The diagnostics of the fava beans anemia can be verified by examination of the level of enzyme G6PD.

The severity of the symptoms and the potential of repercussions are related to the low level of the enzyme. The return of the enzyme level to its normal level is a sign of recovery.

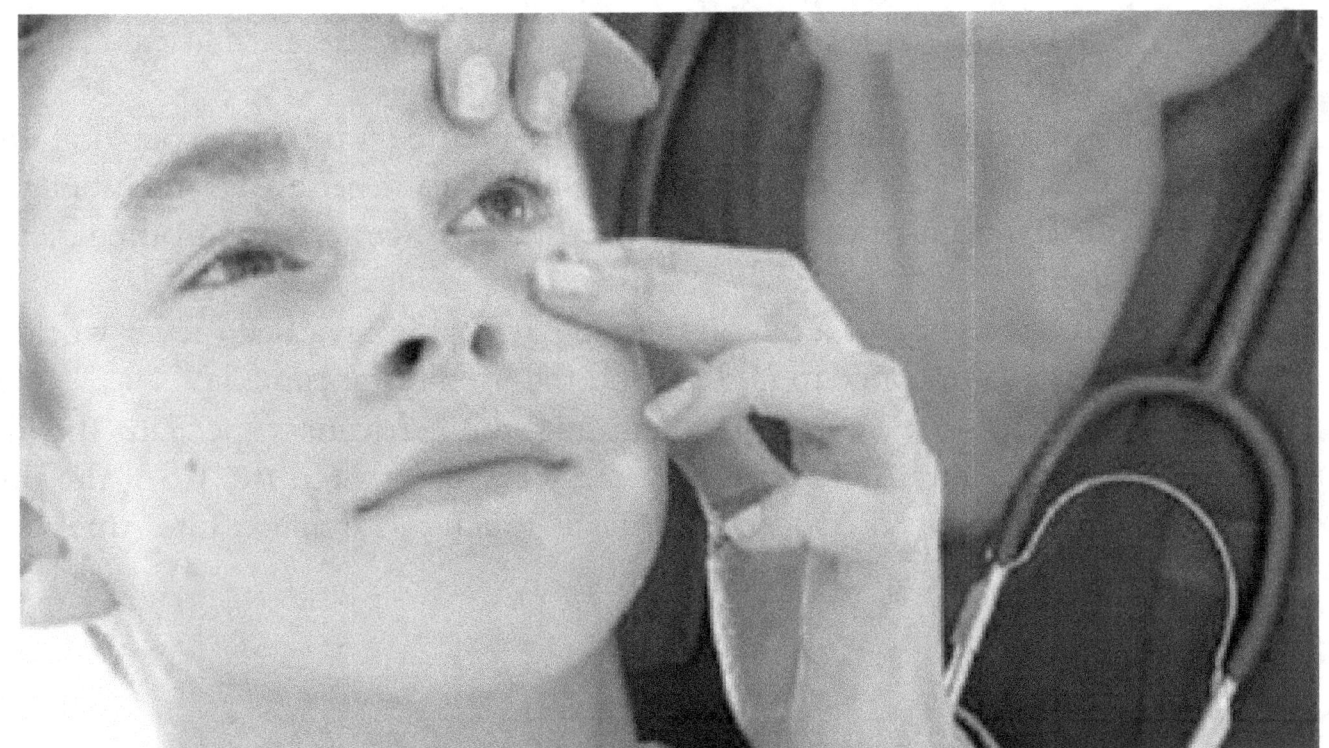
Yellowing of the eye whites is one of the symptoms of the fava bean anemia

Does the Fava Beans Anemia Haunt the Affected Child?

The disease will stay with the sick child throughout the first few years. After reaching 9 to 10 years of age, the body usually starts to gradually produce the enzyme G6PD and replenish the deficit in the enzyme. The level of the enzyme will reach the required level over time and the child will return to health. Usually this will happen upon reaching 20 years of age. It is also possible to follow up the progress by periodically testing the level of the enzyme.

Hereditary Role

- ❖ Gender: The disease transfer by inheritance through a recessive gene on a chromosome X. Since the male has only one of type X while he carries a pair of different chromosomes XY, the disease affects males only and will rarely affect females. On the other hand, the female curies a pair of the chromosome X, that is XX. In this case a good chromosome a defect in the other chromosome. In this case the female may carry the disease but will not contract it.
- ❖ The chance of inheriting the disease by the offsprings increases by marriage of close relatives since the likelihood of having two defective genes increases and that defective gene will be dominant. Therefore, the

medical examination before marriage is important. In that exam the level of the enzyme can be assessed in each party.

- ❖ The defective gene spreads among the members of some specific families. Alternatively, a mutation may take place to a gene of a member of the family without prior spread of the defective gene among other members of the family.
- ❖ There are over half a billion people having the fava bean fever worldwide. The cases are concentrated around the Mediterranean Sea.
- ❖ Race: The disease is spread among the Africans especially the desert dwellers. Many African women carry the disease. In the USA, the disease is spread between African Americans much more than white Americans.

HEREDITARY PROTEIN DISEASE (PKU)

What does PKU Mean?

The name of the disease is Phenylketonuria (PKU) which indicates the seepage of the phenyl ketone with the urine.

In this hereditary disease, there is animosity between the body and the protein. More precisely, a type of amino acids that is considered as the main building blocks of the protein. This type of amino acid is phenylalanine which the body cannot process through metabolism because of the lack of an enzyme necessary for that. The enzyme is phenylalanine hydroxylase. Accordingly, the amino acid accumulates and its level in the blood rises. Subsequently, the Phenyl Ketonuria (P K U) rises in the urine.

Symptoms

The symptoms of that defect in metabolism appear among newborn after consuming a protein that contain the amino acid, such as that present in synthesized milks. They may be delayed in appearance until a few months later after consuming other meals that contain protein. The severity of the symptoms differs according to the extent of the defect.

Generally, there are symptoms and distinguished characteristics of the child who suffers from such defect, such as:

- The child maybe was born underweight.
- The mother notices that her child growing slower than expected.
- The child has thin hair and thin skin that is subject to eczema.
- Microcephaly
- Heart defects
- The accumulation of the amino acid makes the child smell a pungent odor.
- Musty smell.

The lack of metabolism of the amino acid affect the brain activity. In this case, the child suffers from cramps, behavior disorder, and intellectual disability.

What is the Cause of this Brain Imbalance?

To understand the cause of the brain imbalance we have to know the behavior of the amino acid inside the body through the natural metabolism of that amino acid wherein it is converted to tyrosine by the enzyme phenylalanine hydroxylase. The tyrosine is an amino acid used by the brains to produce dopamine, which is a chemical compound necessary for the safety of brain activity.

Those steps do not take place in the presence of defect.

Role of Heredity

- The gene connected to this defect is autosomal recessive and is inherited by both males and females.
- In order for the children to acquire such defect both parents have to be carriers for the defective gene. In this case, the percentage of infecting the son or daughter is about 25% and the percentage of carrying the disease gene by either one is 50%. For this reason, the marriage from close relatives is not recommended due to the increase of the chance of the presence of the defective gene in both. Otherwise a gene examination must be performed for both.
- The disease spreads in the Western countries and the USA more than in Eastern countries. Therefore, some countries conduct blood tests for that amino acid.
- The disease rarely infect African Americans compared to white Americans and other races.
- The percentage of infection by such defect is one in every 12 thousand.
- That defect is connected to the gene PAH which may undergo mutation in one of the family members and it may not be spreading among the previous generations of the same family.
- This specific gene is connected to the enzyme necessary for the metabolism of the amino acid.

Following the Case of a Child

To diagnose this disease, it is necessary to perform blood tests to find out the level of the amino acid phenylalanine. The test should be done periodically for the child to show the levels.

Treatment

There is no treatment that wipes out the defect. Accordingly, the mother has no resort other than putting limitations on the amount of protein in the child's diet. This means reduction in meat, chicken, beans, milk and dairy products. It may also be necessary to watch out for that amino acid that could be present in some artificial sweeteners such as aspartame.

For nursing babies, it is advisable to use special milks free from that amino acid with supplements by small quantities from the mother's milk.

Accordingly, the child must depend in his food regiment to a great extent on vegetables and fruits, in addition to low-protein meals. It is interesting that there are cookbooks for preparation of such meals, written by members from families suffering from heredity defect.

CHANCES OF CONTRACTING ASHKENAZI JEWS DISEASES

Who are the Ashkenazi?

The Ashkenazi are the Jews who have settled in western Europe, as in France and Germany since the Roman Empire. In other words, the Ashkenazi Jews are the Western Jews in contrast with the Mizrahi Jews who are the Eastern Jews and the Sephardi Jews or Spanish Jews.

There are some diseases that were spread among the Ashkenazi and transferred to their children generation after generation and became almost restricted on them. However, these diseases are present on a limited scale, in other places such as the US.

Since the diseases associated with the Ashkenazi are dangerous, have no treatment and can lead to early death the Ashkenazi are subject to genetic survey to prevent the transfer of such diseases to their offsprings.

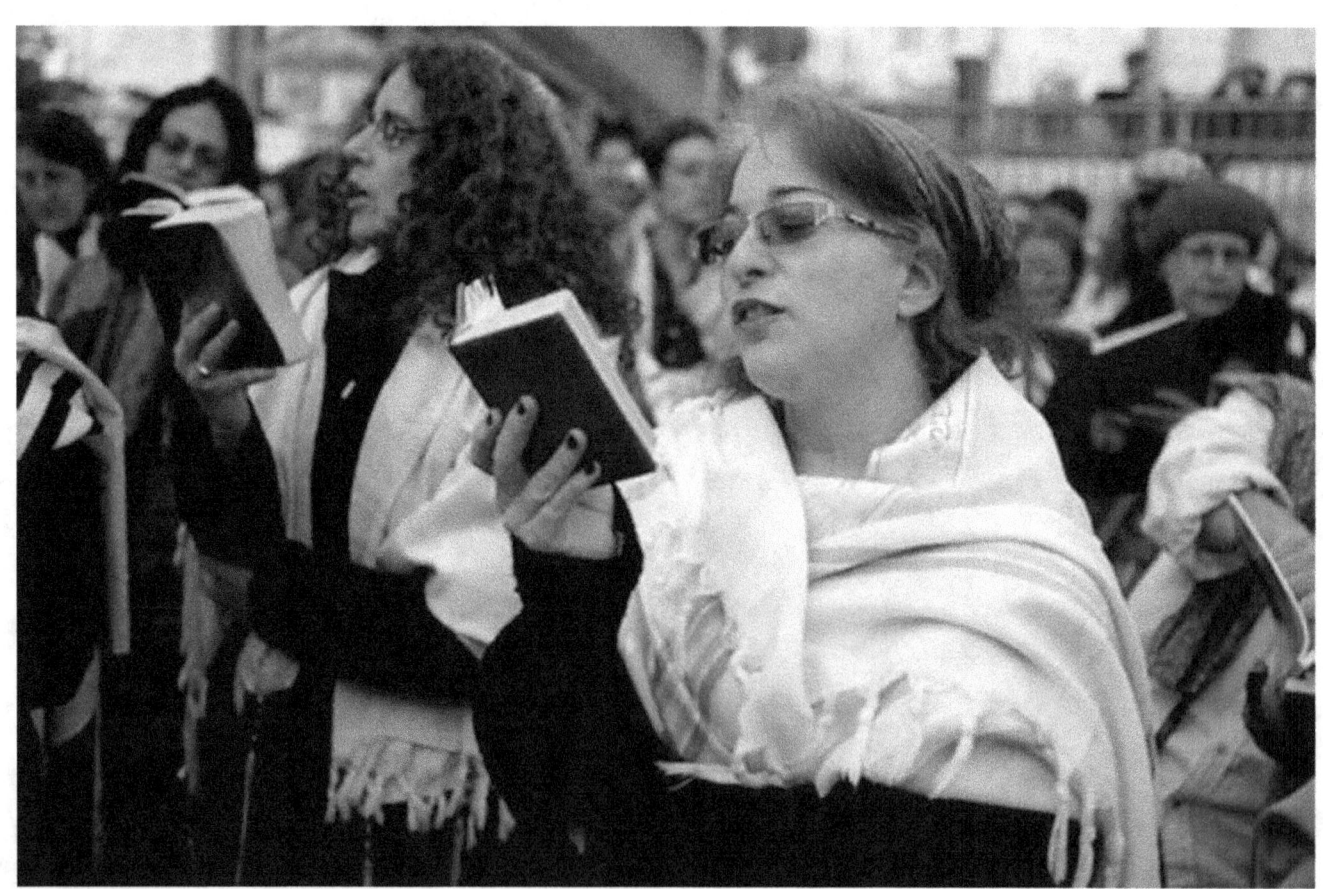

The Ashkenazi

Why did Some Diseases Spread among the Ashkenazi?

Some diseases were spread among the Ashkenazi Jews because of genetic mutation that took place hundreds of years ago due to the intermarriage among them.

The gene carriers do not show the symptoms of the diseases. However, the intermarriage has caused to the appearance of such diseases among their children and grandchildren.

The Most Prominent Diseases

Gaucher Disease

Gaucher's disease or Gaucher disease (GD) is a disease was first recognized by the French doctor Phillippe Gaucher who originally described it in 1882 and lent his name to the condition.

The ratio of occurrence of GD is 1 to 10; that is each ten persons have one of them carrying that disease. The GD has three types the most spread of them is responsive for treatment and is connected to an identified gene, GBA1.

In this type, the genetic disorder is in the shortage of the glucosylceramide enzyme which is needed to digest a fat chemical compound known as a sphingolipid, also known as glucosylceramide.

The glucocerebroside accumulates in cells and certain organs causing health problems in the spleen, liver and bone marrow.

Accordingly, the symptoms of GD are:
- Swelling of the liver.
- Swelling of the spleen.
- Disorder in production of the blood cells from the bone marrow, leading to reduction in the white blood cells and problems related to clotting.

The GD can be treated by Enzyme Replacement Therapy.

Cystic Fibrosis

Cystic Fibrosis is an inherited life-threatening disorder that damages the lungs and digestive system spread at a ratio of one into 24.

Cystic fibrosis affects the cells that produce mucus, sweat, and digestive juices. It causes these fluids to become thick and sticky. They then plug up tubes, ducts, and passageways.

Symptoms vary and can include cough, repeated lung infections, inability to gain weight, and fatty stools.

Treatments may ease symptoms and reduce complications. However, it has no cure and lead to early death usually at the end of thirties. Newborn screening helps with early diagnosis.

Spinal Muscular Atrophy

Spinal Muscular Atrophy (SMA) is connected to the bone marrow and it occurs to one of 41 from the Ashkenazi.

SMA occurs due to reduction in the motor neurons in the bone marrow and the brains stem. Thus, it affects the control of the muscles which shrink with time. There are varieties of the disease and generally, it cannot be treated.